The Mysterious Mind

How to Use Ancient Wisdom and Modern Science to Heal Your Headaches and Reclaim Your Health

By Trupti Gokani, MD

This book does not provide medical, psychiatric, or psychological diagnosis, treatment, or advice. It is for informational purposes only. The dietary and nutritional recommendations described in this book are not intended to substitute for medical advice. Never disregard medical, psychiatric, or psychological advice or treatment and never delay in seeking it because of anything you read in this book. Any questions that you may have regarding the diagnosis or treatment of a medical condition or any product or supplement described in this book should be directed to a qualified healthcare professional.

All matters concerning your health require ongoing medical supervision. If you have a known or suspected medical, psychiatric, or psychological condition, or are taking medications or supplements of any kind, you should consult a qualified healthcare professional before following any of the suggestions described in this book. Any dosages described in this book are intended only as guidelines. You need to consult with your healthcare professional before you use any suggestions found in this book.

The author does not warrant that this book or any information contained in it can be relied upon for applicability to any purpose or treatment, including those described in this book as typical applications for any given supplement or product. With respect to any supplements or products described in this book, the author disclaims any and all warranties, either expressed or implied, including fitness for a particular purpose.

All characters and testimonials provided in this book are either fictitious or have been altered to protect the corresponding patients' identities. Therefore, any resemblance to real persons, or their health conditions or treatments, is purely coincidental.

First edition, April 2015
ISBN: 978-0-692-37842-7

Library of Congress Control Number: 2015935602

Printed in the United States of America

To all of my wonderful patients, many of whom have stood by my side over the years while I evolved and created a new way of practicing headache medicine and treating complex neurological symptoms. I feel blessed that you have shared your wisdom of pain with me, shared your struggles, and shared your glorious moments. I truly thank you for allowing me to share your world. You have been brave even when the pain or symptoms have been unbearable. This book is for you, in hopes of encouraging others to continue to seek approaches and solutions to rid headache pain and other symptoms forever. You deserve that and more.

Table of Contents

Preface

"Either write something worth reading or do something worth writing."
Benjamin Franklin

We are all driven to find purpose and meaning in life. Many of us are put into difficult situations where we are left to either find the meaning and grow from the experience or become disgruntled with the situation and frustrated with the process. Whether we want this to continue or not, life will continue to give us experiences until we fully learn the meaning behind them and grow as individuals. The beauty of aging is that we become wiser. A few gray hairs and wrinkles are definitely worth the wisdom of aging. It is futile to tell ourselves that we wish we had the knowledge we have now when we were younger. We were not supposed to have this knowledge because inherent in these life experiences is a message of personal growth. This is how I view migraines, sleep disorders, depression, anxiety — basically any symptom that presents itself often and repeatedly. Listen to your body; it is telling you something. This language may be challenging to decipher at first, but with time you will fully understand what it is saying.

This book offers you, the sufferer, guidance from a source who has treated individuals using both Western and Eastern approaches. I have embodied the Western approach of utilizing medications and injections and have even recommended surgery, while also delving into the ancient healing principles of Ayurveda. This journey has not been easy for me, but it has been beyond rewarding. We have created a strategy for you to look at your symptoms and find the true meaning behind those symptoms. We will guide you to an understanding that very few will be able to offer. Enjoy the journey and allow yourself to grow and learn.

Trupti Gokani, MD, & the Zira Mind and Body Team
Board-Certified Neurologist, Speaker, Ayurvedic Wellness Coach
Founder, Zira Mind and Body Center

PART I:
Uncover the Mystery

CHAPTER 1
Introduction

"The mass of men lead lives of quiet desperation."
Henry David Thoreau

When most people hear the word "disease," they think of something deadly, uncontrollable and swift — like cancer. But we're facing an epidemic of "dis-ease" — of Americans simply feeling unwell and unable to embrace the lives they want to lead. They're tired, overweight, and inflamed. They are dealing with ongoing digestive issues like constipation or diarrhea (or both), and they aren't sleeping well. And many are suffering from regular headaches — sometimes debilitating ones that impact their ability to enjoy time with family and friends or to devote to their careers.

"I just don't feel healthy," you might say. You look at yourself in the mirror and think, "What happened to the strong, vibrant person I was in my teens, 20s, 30s? Where has she gone and how do I get her back?"

Getting back to a *healthy you* requires that you understand your natural state. Only when you know what a balanced self looks like can you identify the symptoms of imbalance and make appropriate changes to reverse the trajectory of poor health. In ancient Ayurvedic medicine, these natural states come in three kinds called Doshas: Vata, Pitta and Kapha. Your Dosha is the key to your health. And this book will help you identify it and make meaningful change to your life so you can be strong, pain-free and healthy again.

So whether your primary health complaint is your head pain, or you suffer from many seemingly disconnected health symptoms and you are ready to finally understand how it all fits together — how the mysterious mind impacts the entire body and how the magnificent body impacts the mind — this book is for you. Read it cover to cover or jump around among the chapters as they fit your needs and interests. Dr. Gokani's insights, told here in her own words, are bound to awaken a new sense of understanding of your own health, which is the first step in your healing and your happiness.

As a board-certified neurologist specializing in headache pain and neuropsychiatric disorders, I use an integrative medical approach that bridges modern science with an ancient medical practice known as Ayurveda — pronounced ***I-yur-vay-dah.*** As a result, I have helped thousands of patients to overcome debilitating and crippling headache pain and other complex neurological symptoms. I decided to add Ayurveda to my existing traditional model to offer patients a more profound understanding of why they were suffering and what they could do to proactively improve their condition.

Ayurvedic medicine is a system of healing that originated 5,000 years ago in India. The ultimate goal of Ayurveda, which means "science of life," is to guide you in making healthy choices based on the specific needs of your body and mind. You don't have to become a vaidya (an Ayurvedic doctor) to understand the information I am going to share with you. During this journey, it is essential that you remain open to learning something new about yourself and be willing to explore a novel approach to strengthen your mind by strengthening your body.

The key to success in this process is you — it begins with having respect for your own potential to heal and be whole. As your "detective" in unraveling the mystery of your pain and discomfort, I am honored to help you investigate your body's clues and to share the action steps needed to restore your health and close the case on your suffering. But it will be up to you to take action.

Understanding the Roots of Imbalance

We now know that one of the main causes of imbalance and disease is the inability to manage chronic stress on a physical and emotional level. Eating inflammatory foods, suppressing feelings, living a sedentary lifestyle, and grappling with intense work, school, or family situations can all take their toll. Years of imbalance can lead to internal damage and disharmony, causing the mind and body to react with many disease processes, including chronic migraines, ADHD, and mood disorders, for example.

However, the body and mind also have amazing and expansive capacities for healing, especially when provided with the right tools. The Ayurvedic philosophy and lifestyle program is one such tool that I've found to be very effective in mitigating and relieving the cause of headaches and many other symptoms with which you may be contending.

Remember the time you sought advice from your medical doctor because you weren't feeling well? To your surprise, the tests your doctor ordered yielded negative results. I want to assure you that the feeling of discomfort you experienced wasn't your imagination — but it wasn't significant enough to register on traditional diagnostic tests, which are likely only positive when there's at least a 40% breakdown in the body. However, the imbalance at the root of the symptoms was real.

Ayurveda encompasses a broad spectrum of diagnostic tools that makes it possible to recognize and correct this imbalance in its earliest stages. The first step is the determination of your constitutional, or dosha type — Vata, Pitta, or Kapha. The determination of dosha is based on an assessment that includes such factors as complexion and quality of the skin, prominence and shape of joints, body structure, shape of the eyes, manner of walking and talking, weather preferences, and sleeping habits. This assessment, in conjunction with checking radial (wrist) pulses and the condition of the tongue, provides information about the state of the body and mind long before the disease process registers as "positive" on conventional diagnostic tests.

We'll discuss in detail the concept of doshas — and their role as a major clue in the mystery of your migraines and health issues — throughout the course of this book. But first, I'd like to share with you the story of a young patient who struggled with a puzzling health issue that baffled conventional doctors and specialists — and how Ayurvedic practices were the key to solving his mystery.

Kyle's Story

Kyle came to my office with his mother for a consultation. This sweet, happy, and smart young boy was suffering with something that most of us could not even bear for an hour, let alone a day. His symptoms had been occurring daily and persistently for almost two years. Here is his story, as told by his mother.

"My son Kyle began to experience visual distortions and hallucinations in 2011, at the age of seven. Within a span of 10 seconds, the heads of people seemingly changed in size from tiny to gigantic. He called them 'bobble heads.' This was extremely disturbing; he constantly had difficulty looking individuals in the eyes as the change in head size would make him uneasy and nervous, especially with larger groups and classroom settings. Kyle also said the walls around him 'crumbled like paper' and were in constant motion, and sometimes the ground would shift, suddenly forming a V-shaped canyon.

"As I was to later learn, Kyle's visual distortions and hallucinations were consistent with the migraine variant known as Alice In Wonderland Syndrome (AIWS). The following is the clinical description, as published online by the National Institutes of Health:

> *The Alice in Wonderland Syndrome includes an array of symptoms involving altered perception of shape (meta-morphopsia) of objects or persons who appear to be smaller (micropsia) or larger (macropsia) than normal, of impaired sense of passage of time, of zooming of the environment.*[1]

"Within a year, Kyle began experiencing an additional distortion — the horizon began rapidly tilting left to right. My son's experience was even more traumatic because the symptoms were constant instead of intermittent, like most people afflicted with AIWS.

"The journey to search for the cause of these disabling symptoms was long and arduous. Kyle was seen by a broad and vast array of highly-regarded specialists, from pediatric neurologists to pediatric geneticists, in an attempt to accurately diagnose and alleviate the symptoms. Kyle had dozens of appointments and several hospital stays. These doctors ordered a plethora of tests: blood tests, MRIs, MRA, several EEGs, an overnight V-EEG, an EKG, and a lumbar puncture. They administered an IV-magnesium drip and collected several stool samples. Kyle underwent a colonoscopy and endoscopy in search of cancerous tumors. He saw a pediatric rheumatologist to rule out vasculitis as the source of the problem. Kyle also had his eyes examined and refracted several times by an ophthalmologist to ensure the distortions weren't being caused by his vision. He was even seen by a pediatric dentist, who took a full jaw x-ray to make sure the problem didn't stem from Kyle's teeth or jaw alignment. The doctors turned over every stone possible, but they were still unable to determine why Kyle's symptoms were constant, let alone determine how to prevent further progression.

"During this time, Kyle was unable to attend school, play on his sports teams, or attend regular childhood events such as birthday parties. The symptoms were chronic and debilitating, making it a challenge for him to be outside of our home, and his condition significantly impacted our family's life. Still, I was inspired by Kyle's incredible resilience and coping skills. After missing half of the first grade we started homeschooling him and he began to enjoy regular 7-year-old activities, even though the visual distortions were still constant. Somehow, my son had taught himself how to navigate in his 'new world.'

"In early 2012, we applied for the National Institutes of Health's Undiagnosed Diseases Program. The doctors who ran the program were very interested in Kyle's case, and it was under review with their team for nearly nine months. In the end, however, they declined to accept Kyle into the program because they didn't think they could resolve it. Considering all of the tests already conducted and the renowned doctors already consulted, they didn't believe they could add to the findings or help to change Kyle's condition. Their decision was a heavy blow; at the time we believed it was the best — and perhaps the last — option to help our son.

"In the interim, Kyle had devised his own mechanisms to deal with life. His ability to handle the visual distortions was so amazing; the people who didn't know about his condition couldn't tell that he was experiencing anything out of the ordinary. Unfortunately, we knew the truth of his suffering and we wanted it to end more than anything. As his mother, it was agonizing to watch Kyle have to work so hard just to get through the day.

"After two years of constant AIWS symptoms, a friend recommended that we take Kyle to see a neurologist named Dr. Trupti Gokani. My friend said that Dr. Gokani specialized in treating migraine headaches but was also versed in treating other complicated conditions.

"During that first session with her, we shared the whole story — everything Kyle had endured and was presently experiencing. Despite the rare and unconventional nature of Kyle's AIWS symptoms, Dr. Gokani was enthusiastic about finding a way to help our son. As a board-certified neurologist, she was familiar with and fully understood Kyle's clinical situation and the flood of tests and treatments he had already braved. But she also had something else to offer — Ayurvedic medicine. At that time, we had no previous experience with Ayurveda or with any other alternative medical or healing practices. We approached this experience with an open mind and heart, hoping that it would bring Kyle some relief. I am sure you can understand, given our previous journey, why our expectations were tempered.

"We began following the regimen Dr. Gokani prescribed, which included taking an array of herbal supplements and spore-based probiotics, along with making some Ayurvedic lifestyle adjustments. After only six weeks, Kyle experienced his first positive breakthrough in nearly two years! The most debilitating of his visual distortions — the enlarged heads, which made every person around him seem deformed — suddenly stopped. I will never forget the moment when this occurred. We were driving in our car when suddenly Kyle yelled out, 'Mom, your head is not changing in size!' I was in such utter disbelief that I almost swerved off the road. Imagine suffering from that symptom for almost two years, believing it would never go away, and then it suddenly stops! Kyle is nearly 10 now, and we are continuing our work with Dr. Gokani and the Ayurvedic system of healing. We have great hopes for Kyle's full recovery."

Upon follow-up with Kyle's mom, a beautiful ending to a challenging experience was achieved. Kyle, on the day of his birthday, wished for a final resolution of his symptoms. Kyle took a deep breath and blew out his candles with this wish on his mind. On June 13, 2014, a day after his birthday, the syndrome finally ended. Was the emotional mind ready to release what the physical body was holding? We will never know. The mind is a powerful thing; we do know that. In some cases, it is that final will to heal that allows the body to finally be free of symptoms.

Let's Get Started

Kyle's story illustrates how even a mystery as extreme and debilitating as his may be solved through Ayurvedic practices and integrative healing. Are you ready to solve the mystery of your own ailments and enjoy your life free from pain and distress? Good news — the path to relief begins as soon as you turn the page!

Part I of this book, "Uncover the Mystery," introduces you to a surprising and simple way to think about your health. You'll discover that the mind is a mysterious machine with a complex relationship with the rest of the body, and that integrative healing — the coupling of conventional medicine and Ayurvedic principles — facilitates mind-body balance, allowing you to treat the underlying causes of your pain and not just its symptoms.

Part II, "Investigate the Clues," unravels several important clues that are fundamental to understanding and identifying your body's unique composition and what causes your imbalance. You'll learn about your body's biochemistry, discover how digestion and adrenal function are the master keys to health, and take the dosha assessment test to determine your dominant dosha and then examine its characteristics in depth.

Part III, "Close the Case," presents action steps and tools for restoring balance to your mind and body in order to reverse the trajectory of poor health. You'll find recommendations for meaningful dietary and lifestyle changes, as well as information on conventional medications and nutritional supplements.

Mind-body balance is the key to vibrant well-being and longevity and is the ultimate goal of my recommended protocol. It is my hope that this book will help you achieve that goal and experience the joy of optimal health.

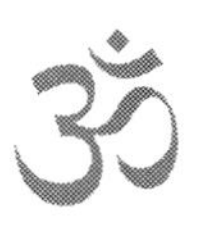

CHAPTER 2
The Mysterious Mind Deciphered

"Biology gives you a brain. Life turns it into a mind."
Jeffrey Eugenides

As we uncover the mystery of the mind-body relationship, you'll find that my neurological perspective is layered in Eastern medicine. I use Ayurvedic medicine in conjunction with conventional medical protocols (often referred to as Western or allopathic medicine) because I firmly believe this combination is the best of both worlds. I reached this conclusion after a 10-year journey, which I share with you in the next chapter. From firsthand experience, I've found Ayurveda to be an exceptional, complementary approach to healthcare. Conventional medicine provides pain relief, while Ayurvedic assessments help you reconnect to your body's unique needs and ideal state of balance. You also benefit from the Ayurvedic approach because it helps you understand why you have health issues and migraine headaches, and it leads to a decrease in the overall number of occurrences.

The success I've experienced in treating many forms of pain is based on the premise that all symptoms are potentially a manifestation of multiple systems gone awry, rather than a single system experiencing dysfunction. Combining conventional and Ayurvedic principles helps individuals to understand the underlying causes, rather than just treating the symptoms. No matter how long the problem has been manifesting, based on the principles of Ayurvedic medicine the root cause is always the same — imbalance. This imbalance can manifest in your structure, physiology, psychology, or all three. You must determine the cause of the systemic imbalance so that it can be corrected.

Ayurvedic philosophy teaches that balance is fostered when your body, mind, and spirit are in harmony with nature. This harmony can be achieved by doing something as simple as creating a regular routine for going to bed and awakening, eating foods that nourish the body, or exercising in a way that is best for your unique type. In *Healing Through Ayurveda*, author Sonica Krishan further explains why this is important:

> *Like nature, we're made up of the five basic elements: ether (aakasha), air (vayu), fire (tejas), water (jala), and earth (prithvi). Ether represents the empty space between the body organs, inside the ears, in the minute cells, etc. The air element imparts all the movement that we experience like breathing, blinking of the eyes, working of the body organs, and mobility. Fire in the body represents metabolic heat, gastric heat, body temperature. Water is present in the form of saliva, blood, plasma, various secretion and digestive juices. Earth makes up all the matter within us, like muscles, bones, tendons, ligaments, and everything else that adds to the body substance. The balance of the five elements is different in everyone. From the time of birth, these elements merge in various proportions resulting in varied bodily persona and mental traits.*[2]

Further, Ms. Krishan writes, "Ayurvedic medicine sees you as rhythmic as the seasons, as powerful as the stars, as ageless as time because you are made up of the same dynamic elements that compose the cosmos."[3]

Conventional medicine looks at the structure of the body, while Ayurvedic medicine takes into account the energy behind the physical structure. According to Ayurvedic principles, there are three different types of energy — known as doshas — that govern the functions in the mind and body. These doshas represent the physical and mental characteristics inherent in all people:

- Vata (a combination of air and space elements)
- Pitta (a combination of fire and water elements)
- Kapha (a combination of water and earth elements)

Depending upon your dosha, your system has definable digestive capabilities; you have a unique mind type and a specific body physique, as well as distinctive headache presentations.

Conventional medical researchers have just begun to understand what Ayurvedic and Chinese medical doctors have always known to be true — the body is an interconnected organism, and this interconnection

Three Ayurvedic Types (Figure 1)

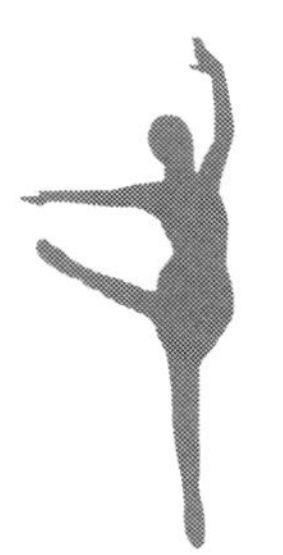

Vata
(A combination of air and space elements. Thin in physical stature. An artist.)

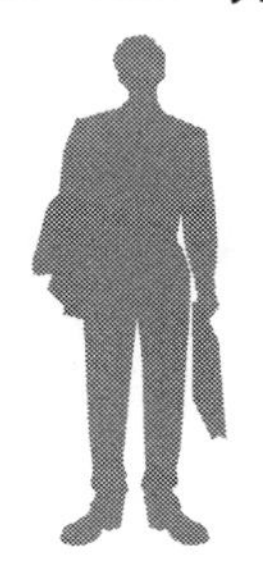

Pitta
(A combination of fire and water elements. Muscular in physical stature. A lawyer.)

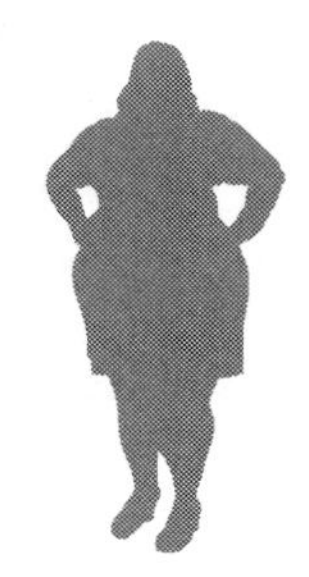

Kapha
(A combination of water and earth elements. Large in physical stature. A homemaker.)

impacts digestion, brain function, hormonal balance, and mood. According to a study published in the *Journal of Headache Pain,* researchers now know that digestive issues are fairly common among patients with migraine headaches; approximately half of them have been found to have symptoms of acid reflux, and 22% have been diagnosed with gastroesophageal reflux disease (GERD).[4]

In a study I conducted examining the prevalence of food intolerances in patients who have migraines, out of 500 patients I found that 59% had moderate to high intolerance reactions after consuming dairy products, 36% had reactions after consuming eggs, 47% had a moderate to high reaction after consuming wheat, and 22% had moderate to high reactions after consuming certain fruits. As a result, I have recommended dietary modifications to avoid food intolerances and have found that this change reduces certain digestive symptoms, fatigue, headaches, and other symptoms. These results also demonstrate how addressing digestive issues first may actually improve neurologic well-being.

A primary principle of Ayurvedic medicine is that all imbalances, illnesses, or chronic diseases (from the sniffles to cancer) begin in a specific location of the body, based on your dosha. Understanding your dosha type provides an immediate gateway to the root cause of illness. For Vata, the imbalance begins in the colon; for Pitta, the imbalance manifests in the small intestines; and for Kapha, the imbalance is expressed in the stomach. Did you notice that each of these organs plays a role in the process of digestion? Even ancient medical protocols recognized the state of one's digestive function as an essential component of health and well-being.

This information has become integral to the development of the treatment protocol I recommend. When I first meet with patients, I often order a series of biochemistry tests. I also seek to determine their most prominent dosha (Vata, Pitta, or Kapha) and work to understand how that dosha is manifesting in both the balanced and imbalanced states. Sometimes patients have been experiencing debilitating pain for so long that they are emotionally disconnected from their balanced state. The treatment protocol is specific and unique to each individual, and it includes dietary changes, herbal remedies, gentle exercise (such as yoga), and getting more rest.

As you learned from my patient Kyle's story, incorporating Ayurveda helps me fine-tune my decisions about which conventional agents are most effective for symptom reduction. An anxious patient with the Vata dosha type, for example, might respond well to a benzodiazepine (such as Valium), while a Pitta dosha type with a headache behind the eyes might respond best to onabotulinumtoxinA (Botox Type A). A person experiencing congestion from an imbalanced Kapha dosha may have success with fexofenadine (Allegra). From an integrative medical perspective, patients often respond better to these conventional medications once their systems are more in balance.

The Mystery of the Migraine

"Migraine is a spiritual intervention from God. When we are afflicted with migraine, it is a sign that we have been too caught up with our worldly affairs and, thus, disconnected with ourselves and the rhythms of nature."

Vasant Lad, B.A.M.S., M.A.Sc, Ayurvedic Physician — NAMA Conference 2008

I will never forget sitting in the audience listening to Dr. Vasant Lad. He had just given one of the most powerful lectures I had ever heard about migraine headaches. Although the diagnosis of migraine is still one of the most misunderstood phenomena in medicine, calling it a "spiritual intervention" seemed like a radical comparison. I was certain very few of my patients would fathom referring to migraine headaches as "spiritual interventions." These disabling attacks of pain, which have been linked to a neurological storm of nausea, sensitivities, and mood symptoms often left the sufferer exhausted, frustrated, and apprehensive about the next episode. Yet Dr. Lad's description motivated me to probe more deeply into the Ayurvedic assessment of migraines.

According to Dr. Lad, descriptions of migraine headaches were found in ancient Ayurvedic texts. In Ayurveda, this type of headache was referred to as *Ardhaavabheda*. *Ardhaava* means "half side of the head" and *vabheda* means "breaking pain." While the etymology of the word "migraine" has been linked to French, Latin, and Greek cultures, it's interesting to note that the translations are similar to the Ayurvedic: "pain on one side of the head."

The exact origins or causes of "pain on one side of the head" are often a mystery. Conventional medicine developed its own classification system of migraine headaches, which include the following characteristics:

- Moderate to severe in intensity
- Lasting a few hours to a few days
- Association with nausea and/or vomiting
- Light and sound sensitivity
- Pulsating in nature
- Usually occurring on one side
- Aggravated by routine physical activity
- Triggers aren't always consistent and clear, but involve exposure to fluctuations in hormones, weather, stress, and certain foods
- About 20-30% of patients may have an "aura," which is a visual and/or sensory phenomenon that can precede an attack of pain
- Women are impacted three times more often than men

After more than a decade of working with people experiencing the pain of migraine headaches, I have accumulated the skills, information, and knowledge to help my patients alleviate and, in some cases, totally eradicate the symptoms. But before you get too excited, it's important to know that this change doesn't occur overnight. In fact, it can take weeks, months, and possibly even years for there to be a *sustainable* difference. However, if you're willing to do the work and make some alterations in your lifestyle and your approach to these attacks, I am confident that you will achieve long-lasting, positive results!

The Six Stages of Disease[5]

Ayurvedic medicine is based on the principle that there are six stages of the disease process.

Stage 1: **Accumulation** begins in an organ of one of the three main dosha sites when excessive lifestyle choices, such as too much stress or too much fast food, lead to an internal blockage. Minor symptoms are noted at this step, such as gas (Vata), heartburn (Pitta), or bloating (Kapha).

Stage 2: **Aggravation** occurs when accumulation continues without treatment. The symptoms become more bothersome, last longer, and occur more frequently.

Stage 3: **Dissemination** results when the imbalance in the original organ of the aggravated dosha increases beyond capacity. Symptoms become more pronounced.

Stage 4: **Localization** occurs when the aggravation spreads to weaker organs of the dosha (i.e., inflammation in the digestive system leads to an inflamed right knee, without symptoms of pain).

Stage 5: **Manifestation** is the first stage in which conventional or Western medical tests can discern a sign of disease. The disorder is now fully developed with clinical features (i.e., right knee is now painful).

Stage 6: **Disruption** is the chronic stage. It occurs when a person ignores the previous symptoms. Now the illness shows signs that help identify its dosha origin, and there may be complications as well. Healing from chronic illness is possible, but it takes the longest to achieve (i.e., right knee pain and right side of the head are now painful).

During Stages 1 and 2, making dietary shifts and lifestyle adjustments can reverse the imbalance in most cases. In Stages 3 and 4, the Ayurvedic protocol often includes herbal therapies and cleansing procedures. In Stages 5 and 6, multiple approaches are needed to address the physical and mental imbalances.

No matter what the symptoms or disease, the great news is that with Ayurveda you have the chance to reverse the process! It's never too late to create conditions for the body to heal. It may require a longer period of time or take more work, but healing can occur. It is during this time that an action plan and realistic goals are needed. All change begins in the mind — making up your mind that you're ready to change is the first and, most often, the hardest step. It can be a baby step if that's all you can fathom at the moment. But I promise that if you take even a baby step, change in your overall health and well-being is bound to occur!

If your condition has been chronic for a long time, it's hard to envision a life without pain or discomfort. It may seem that having days or months without symptoms would be impossible to achieve. I ask that you take a moment and close your eyes. Breathe deeply. Ask yourself: What would my life be like if I didn't have migraine headaches, fatigue, or depression? Who would I be? What would I be doing differently? Jot down your answers. There is no right or wrong response. To move forward you just need a template, and answering the questions in the dosha assessment (Part II) will help you create one. You choose how slowly or quickly you move forward. Remember, healing occurs in phases. I simply encourage you to begin the process.

Who Are You ... Really?

During an initial visit with a neurologist most patients with fatigue, headaches, insomnia, or other symptoms believe the scope of the visit will focus entirely on their headaches or chief complaint. A visit to my office is very different. I ask about non-neurological symptoms such as gas, bloating, and constipation. Most often the patients look surprised and, in turn, I often am surprised by their responses. Many of them share that their history of constipation has been a chronic symptom for years. Some reveal that they only have one bowel movement (or less) per week! It still amazes me that for most of these patients, I am the first physician who has connected the dots between their long history of digestive issues and their current neurological condition (see Chapter 5 for more details).

Without a complete picture of all the symptoms, the ability to diagnose and help you heal is limited. That's why your awareness of the mind-body connection is essential. It helps you develop the ability to recognize when your body is out of balance so that you can employ the dietary, exercise, and stress-reduction tools necessary for creating balance. Balance is the key to helping your body heal. (You'll find more information about this in Part III.)

Imagine that you're having dinner with friends at a nice restaurant and you begin to feel tired. At that moment, you have two choices — you can have another glass of wine and ignore the fact that your mind and body are urging you to go home (after all, you work hard and do not get to see your friends as often as you would like), or you can cordially depart and go home to give your body the rest it is requesting. While you may instinctively know the best choice, too often the quest for pleasure — fueled by food, alcohol, and medication — overrides your ability to clearly hear your body's messages. That's why I believe Ayurveda is the essential component for creating balance so that your body can heal.

One of the primary principles of Ayurveda is that everyone is born with a specific doshic composition. A dosha is your body's unique constitution, comprised of some combination of the five elements of air, space, fire, earth, and water. The three doshas are Vata, Pitta, and Kapha. There is no need to memorize the details; you simply need to become familiar with your specific mind-body type. Knowing your specific dosha type is helpful in order to effectively work toward ridding yourself of those nagging headache symptoms and other symptoms you are experiencing. Remember that it's a system, not a symptom, that we will be treating. Improving one symptom will likely lead to an improvement of another, seemingly-unrelated symptom. Isn't that nice?

As shown in *Figure 1,* individuals with the Vata dosha are primarily composed of air and space elements, those with the Pitta dosha are individuals composed of fire and water elements, and Kapha dosha individuals are composed of earth and water elements. What does this mean? Each dosha has specific digestive capabilities, mind types, body physiques, and headache symptoms.

By understanding your primary dosha, which you will decipher in Part II, you'll begin to see that all symptoms or chronic diseases are an expression of an imbalanced system, or imbalanced dosha. The key to restoring that balance involves identifying your dosha and making dietary adjustments and lifestyle changes, coupled with taking the appropriate supplements. The combination of these factors will lead to the reduction and eventual alleviation of headache symptoms and many other symptoms you may be experiencing.

Vata individuals tend to have a thinner build or smaller bone structure and are often in motion. The combination of air and space elements creates movement and wind. Vata energy controls bodily functions associated with motion, including blood circulation, breathing, blinking, and heartbeat. Take a moment and think about wind blowing through your body. It makes you feel cool and dry. Vata individuals have a tendency to always feel cold, or they may perpetually have cold hands and feet. They also are prone to dry skin and experience internal dryness, which leads to constipation, gas, and bloating. A balanced Vata mind is creative. But when this dosha is out of balance, the individual is prone to anxiety and often has difficulty focusing.

Pitta individuals tend to have a medium build. The energy of Pitta controls the body's metabolic systems (including digestion, absorption, and nutrition) and the body's temperature. Pitta individuals tend to be intelligent, detailed, focused, and driven. They are often perfectionists and can process and "see" things very clearly. They are the first to comment on how things should be done, as they feel they have the best perspective on life. Out of balance, Pitta individuals tend to anger quickly and become critical. They often don't tolerate warm weather or heat.

Individuals with a Kapha dosha tend to have a larger physical frame. The energy of Kapha controls growth in the body. It also supplies water to all body parts, moisturizes the skin, and maintains the immune system. Kapha individuals tend to have relaxed, contemplative personalities and are often quite nurturing and caring. When out of balance, Kapha individuals are prone to congestion and weight gain. They can also struggle with insecurity and depression.

You may find that one of these descriptions perfectly describes your predominant type, or you may find that your constitution is an equal combination of all three doshas. Each of us has all of the elements within us. But at birth, some elements inherently exist at a higher level. Most people with combined doshas do have a primary dosha, and the other

Localization of Excess Energy Based on Doshas (Figure 2)

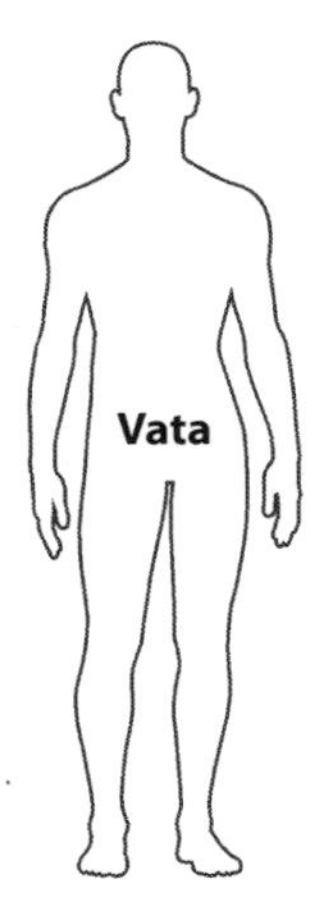

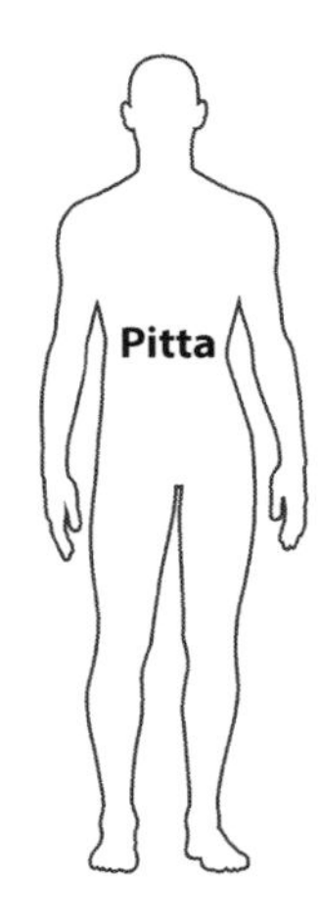

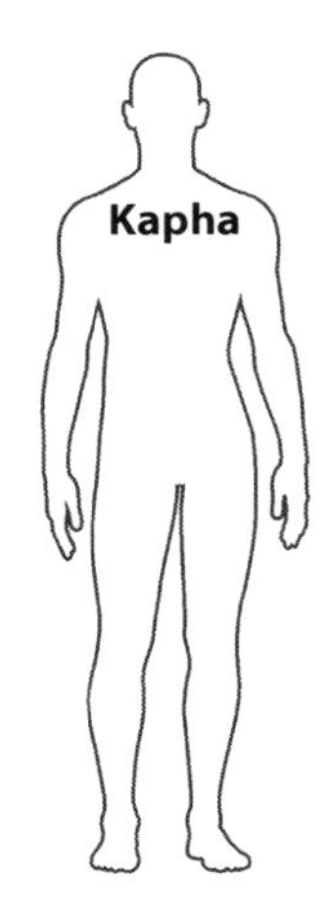

Vata energy localizes to the colon and can lead to gas/bloating/ constipation.

Pitta energy localizes to the small intestine and can lead to indigestion/ burning and nausea.

Kapha energy localizes to the stomach and chest and leads to heaviness and congestion.

characteristics are still important, but play a lesser role in their lives. Your specific dosha or constitutional type will play an integral part in the development of your treatment protocol. You will have an opportunity to participate in a self-assessment to determine your dominant dosha in Part II of this book and, as a result, you will be amazed by how clearly you'll be able to understand what's going on in your body and your life.

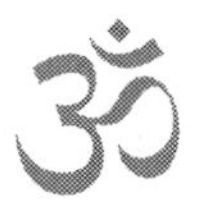

CHAPTER 3
Taking the Road Less Traveled

"Do not go where the path may lead; go instead where there is no path and leave a trail."
Ralph Waldo Emerson

As your "detective" in the quest to close the case on your pain and discomfort, you may be wondering how I arrived in this position. What led me to discover integrative medicine? Why did I choose to seek additional healing options? How did I uncover the mystery of the mind-body relationship? I'd like to share my story with you.

After completing a traditional residency training program in neurology, I began my medical practice working in one of the finest headache centers in the Chicago area. I spent the first few years learning about and prescribing traditional medications used to prevent and terminate migraines. During that time, I decided to complete training in psychopharmacology in order to fully understand how the medications prescribed for migraines worked and how their interaction impacted the human body. I learned to administer trigger-point injections and Botulinum Toxin Type A injections. I also gave many patients referrals for psychotherapy in order to help them deal with the stress of the chronic migraine condition. In short, I was helping my patients manage their pain, but little else.

The more specialized in headaches I became, the more I realized how my approach was reductionist. Looking back, I think this narrowing of focus happens to many doctors who choose to specialize in one area of medicine; their perspective is driven by their area of focus, rather than taking into account how additional factors can impact the whole. Neurologists, for example, believe that the nervous system function is based on the strength of this system alone, and they focus energy on the inner workings of the brain, spinal cord, and all of the nerves in the body. Consequently, the other organs or body systems start to become less important. A problem with the head generally means there is an issue with the brain. The main focus is to create a brain that functions optimally by giving the brain specific attention.

As my practice continued to evolve, I began to zero in on the specific neurotransmitter or inflammatory peptide responsible for the headache and/or mood disorder the patient was experiencing. Like many of my colleagues I believed serotonin, a neurotransmitter that regulates moods, appetite, and sleep, was also involved in migraine generation. Therefore, I focused on the marvelous pharmacological agents that targeted this neurotransmitter, such as the triptans. Those serotonin-receptor agonists are a powerful tool for disabling headaches in many patients.

But despite my focused intent, I had not yet recognized the importance of investigating the cause of the release of these neuroinflammatory peptides or why some patients had low serotonin in the first place. I continued to be baffled by the fact that certain patients had a partial or lack of response to the triptan migraine medications.

After three years at the headache center, I felt dissatisfied; I knew something was missing. It wasn't the work environment or the patients — I was working in a beautiful office with patients who were wonderful. But the discomfort, which I've since grown to trust as my guide, was pushing me to explore the world of pain from a different perspective. This led me to step outside of my comfort zone and open my own clinic. At that moment, however, I had no inkling about the vastly different direction I eventually would take.

The World of Functional Medicine

The first time I heard the term "functional medicine" was during a casual conversation in the hallway of my new headache clinic. At the time, I was sharing office space with a chiropractor who directed a wellness center. He suggested I learn more about it. We then went back to our respective offices. I had absolutely no idea what the term "functional" meant in relation to medicine, but the concept stayed with me. As I was to later learn, functional medicine focuses on the total health and well-being of the patient. It uses a systems-oriented approach in which the doctor focuses on the whole patient, rather than just the symptoms. Integrative medicine combines both Western (traditional) medicine with Eastern (alternative) medicine. Functional medicine goes a step further. This approach involves looking at the "functioning" of the system to see where the body is not functioning optimally. For example, you may complain to your physician about low thyroid symptoms, but your thyroid labs appear normal. A functional practitioner will look at the labs and may find that some of the tests may appear "low normal" in the testing range. This practitioner may even check further labs which are not routine or have you submit urine or saliva samples to obtain a measure of your hormones from a different perspective. Combining this with the clinical symptoms may lead that practitioner to offer a supplement, diet, or even a medication to improve the symptoms and bring the labs to a more optimal range.

Shortly thereafter, I learned about a three-day functional medicine conference. During the very first conference session I learned that in order to have vibrant health, all of the body's systems (such as the digestive, nervous, respiratory, and circulatory) need to efficiently operate in concert. I felt as if I had just been handed the key to understanding how the human body truly functioned. It suddenly became clear to me that a migraine, which was once strictly considered a neurologic condition, could now be traced to any number of conditions, such as digestive imbalances, food allergies, or thyroid dysfunction.

The more I continued my study of the migraine and other neurological symptoms based on this new paradigm, the more I realized how complicated it was for the body's nervous system to independently generate an attack of pain or symptomatology. During a migraine attack, even though an excitable brain and an activated brainstem lead to changes in serotonin activity, this excitability occurs when the system is provoked. The truth is that this activity — along with inflammation of the nerve endings, dilation of cranial blood vessels, and the entire activation of the nervous system — is closely connected to the entire physiology of the body (*see Figure 3*).

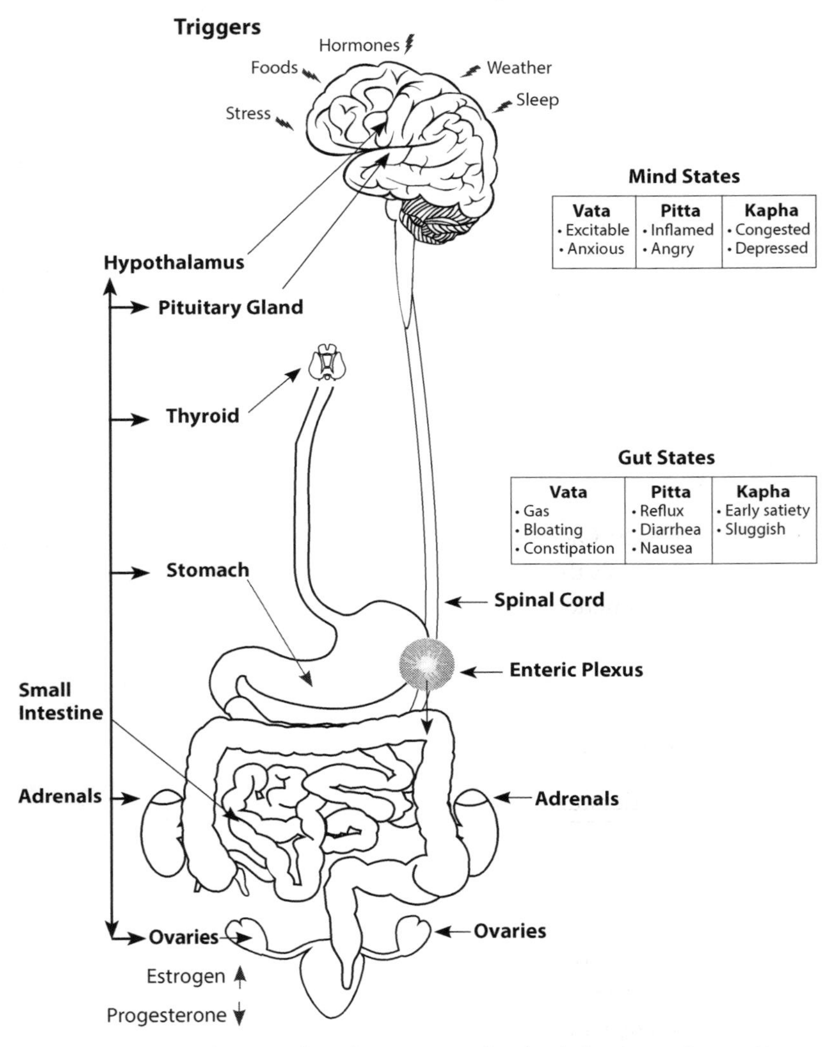

The key to understanding neurological symptoms, such as headaches, insomnia, mood issues and fatigue, is the realization that there is a strong link between the gut and brain. In addition, the nervous system is intimately connected to our adrenal system, ovaries and thyroid gland. When the brain becomes excitable, inflamed and/or congested, it often is a result of the adrenals, ovaries and thyroid system not being in optimal balance. Balancing these organs can strengthen the brain and improve brain function.

The intricate links between the body's organ systems soon became more clear. I began to understand how dysfunction in the digestive tract — poor digestion due to food intolerance, pesticides, or other toxins — impaired the liver and compromised its ability to detoxify. Those accumulated toxins in the liver and in the fatty tissues of the brain caused fatigue, mood changes, and headaches. I soon concluded that the migraine was actually a symptom related to the digestive system and possibly other organ systems, rather than a symptom caused by dysfunction of the brain.

To substantiate my new conclusion, I began scouring my patients' lab tests in search of links to digestive imbalances. The subsequent recommendations I made included dietary changes, exercise, stress reduction, yoga, B vitamin and/or magnesium supplements, or herbal remedies. These powerful and effective interventions could be used in conjunction with conventional care and medications. My goal was to help my patients build a foundation of health that could potentially reduce the need or reliance on pharmaceutical drugs.

The Hippocratic Oath is a code of ethics to which all physicians swear to adhere. It requires that doctors keep their patients from harm, and it is a basic tenet of functional medicine's approach to health. Because many pharmaceutical drugs potentially cause a cascade of secondary issues, the goal in functional medicine is to first rebalance the body naturally, without using medications. One might argue that making dietary changes is potentially a lot less harmful than taking a prescription drug.

The Road to Understanding

The more I employed the functional medicine model — the model of finding the underlying imbalance — the more I sought deeper answers. I pondered why some individuals tended to be more ill than others; I wanted to know who was most prone to disease. Ultimately, I turned to the country of my heritage, India, and began training in Ayurvedic medicine. Finally, I found a system of healing that answered even my most complicated questions about symptoms and disease. Ayurveda offered a precise and unique method of evaluation that I could readily integrate into my practice.

Ayurveda focuses on prevention and healing by teaching how to live in harmony with the basic laws of nature. What are these laws? Let me give you an example: As the sun rises, you should awaken. As the sun sets, you should go to sleep. When your body signals hunger, you should eat. If stressed, you should take steps to relax.

When you look at your day, are you in tune with any of these signals? When you are aware of the signals, do you follow them? Most people do not. Why? Most people are pulled in multiple directions; obligations or personal interests tend to take precedence over their body's needs. The proliferation of internet access, cell phone barrages, late-night TV, and restaurants that offer late-night dinners also afford ample opportunity to ignore the body's most pressing needs.

Ayurveda provided me with tremendous insights on the root causes of both health and disease based on the innate physiological type that we all possess. Using nature as a model helps you reset the body's circadian rhythm which can, when imbalanced, predispose the body to chronic disease. To achieve balance, it's essential that you understand your body's specific needs and then take positive action. In Parts II and III of this book we set out to do just that.

PART II:
Investigate the Clues

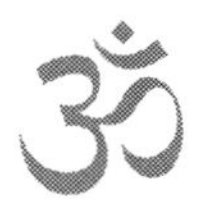

CHAPTER 4
Understanding Your Body's Biochemistry

"A man's mind is stretched by a new idea or sensation, and never shrinks back to its former dimensions."
Oliver Wendell Holmes, Sr.

Western medical doctors review and interpret test results using what are referred to as "laboratory reference range values." Have you ever wondered how the "normal range" is determined? The Clinical and Laboratory Standards Institute provides guidelines and criteria to laboratories around the country for calculating a baseline "healthy reference population." The "healthy population" is based on a specific number of people of different sexes, ages, and races who meet multiple criteria. While each laboratory testing your blood or urine can potentially have its own baseline of "normal," most of these ranges tend to be fairly close among laboratories.[6]

If any of your results are in "normal range," conventional medical doctors will usually give you a clean bill of health. Unfortunately, the most common complaints that precipitate a visit to a doctor, such as fatigue or a chronic headache, often show up in "normal range" on most medical tests. Your doctor will then tell you that you're doing fine, or maybe he or she will give you a prescription for antibiotics "in case you're coming down with something." You know in your heart that your body is not in balance, whether the labs reveal this or not.

The ideal way to review lab results is to determine if you fall into the "optimal" range versus simply falling within the upper and lower limits of normal. The labs also need to be evaluated in a systems-based fashion. One organ may reveal an imbalance if another organ isn't functioning optimally. The optimal goals I present in this chapter were developed after more than a decade of working with thousands of patients.

Learning from Common Laboratory Tests

Let's examine the most commonly ordered laboratory tests and how they may be interpreted when evaluating the state of your health.

Glucose

Normal range: 65-99 mg/dL
Optimal goal: 70-80 mg/dL*

This test measures your blood sugar and is best evaluated during a fasting state. Patients who experience high levels of stress tend to release a higher amount of cortisol during this time, which can lead to elevated blood sugars. This cortisol release can also occur after a high-glycemic meal, such as macaroni and cheese, a bagel made with processed flour (white, wheat, or multigrain), or a piece of chocolate cake.

If your glucose is high (hyperglycemic), dietary changes (such as avoiding grains), undergoing hydration, and engaging in stress-relieving activities (such as yoga, tai chi, walking, meditation, and deep breathing) are essential. It is always wise to increase the amount of green vegetables and healthy fats (from raw nuts to avocados), seeds, and lentils that you eat.

At times, the glucose is below range (hypoglycemic) or on the very low side of normal. This may be the case for patients diagnosed with fibromyalgia or those who have very weak adrenals and low cortisol production. This situation can be addressed with the use of supplements to strengthen the adrenals and by making sure that the system receives nourishment from high-quality foods throughout the day.[7]

Hemoglobin A1C

Normal range: Less than 5.7% of total Hgb
Optimal goal: Less than 5.0% of total Hgb*

This test provides a window of how well-regulated the blood sugars have been over a three month period of time.[8] This number should be monitored closely if you are on progesterone and if you are at risk for diabetes. Also, if there has been an increase in weight, especially around your midsection, this is an important number to review.[9]

If this number is high or increases over time, it is necessary to re-evaluate factors such as the medications you are taking, your exercise program, and adrenal stress, as well as your overall emotional well-being.

Vitamin D, 25 OH, Total (combination of Vit D, 25 OH D2 and D3)

Normal range: 30-100 ng/mL
Optimal goal: 50 ng/mL*

Vitamin D breaks the rules for vitamins because it's produced in the human body, not obtained from food. (It is contained in fish and egg yolks, but it is not bioavailable directly from the ingestion of those foods as Vitamin D.) It's not really a vitamin, but rather a fat-soluble, steroid hormone. Still, it has "vitamin-like" properties. For instance, Vitamin D has been found to support the immune system.[10]

Researchers have also found that Vitamin D becomes depleted under stress, or when the body has low progesterone levels. In addition, low levels of Vitamin D have been linked to obesity, migraines, and bone health, and a host of other conditions. [11]

It is recommended to spend 15-30 minutes daily in the sun — exposing full arms, face, and legs if possible — between the hours of 10 a.m. and 2 p.m. However, this is only effective at helping bodies produce 10,000 IUs of Vitamin D3 between the months of May and September for people living anywhere north of Atlanta.[12]

During the other months, I believe that Vitamin D supplementation is necessary. I recommend a daily dosage of Vitamin D3 between 2,000 IU and 5,000 IU, depending on the body's needs. I also recommend that Vitamin D3 be taken with Vitamin K2, which also helps strengthen bone and has been found to support the cardiovascular system.

Some of my patients have experienced better moods, more energy, and a decline in headaches when their Vitamin D range is closer to 60-70ng/mL. My patient Linda had daily migraines for 28 years, which controlled her life. In 2007, after seeing more than 13 neurologists and taking more than 50 medications over the years, she became my patient. I was able to break the pain cycle with conventional medications, but Linda still continued to have intermittent headaches. When I first learned about the link between Vitamin D3 depletion and migraines, I had Linda tested. Her levels were extremely low. I tried various dosages until she was taking 5,000 IU per day. The migraines ended completely, and she was able to stop taking all of the other conventional medications. In addition, Linda could drink wine, eat chocolate, and dive into her career as an artist at the age of 68!

The Thyroid Gland's Essential Role

The thyroid gland produces hormones that regulate the body's metabolic rate, as well as the heart and digestive function, muscle control, brain development, and bone maintenance. It also modulates the body's temperature. Although researchers aren't fully aware of all the reasons, we do know that the thyroid's delicate balance is essential when attempting to overcome migraine headaches. I pay acute attention when looking at the final test results, which may require my patients to take additional medications or nutritional supplements.

Thyroid Stimulating Hormone (TSH)

Normal range: 0.50-4.0 mIU/L
Optimal goal: 0.50-2.0 mIU/L*

The thyroid stimulating hormone (TSH) is produced by the hypothalamus (our circadian pacemaker) to inform the thyroid gland about the body's thyroid hormone status. Often TSH can become suppressed due to stress. When reviewing the tests, we sometimes see low thyroid hormone and low TSH. When this is the case, I look at RT3 (reverse T3) as a true gauge of what is happening with the thyroid. Iodine status can also influence TSH. Patients suffering from headaches who may also have thyroid issues generally complain of fatigue, weight gain, "foggy brain," hair loss, constipation, and/or brittle nails.[13, 15]

T4 (Thyroxine), Total

Normal range: 4.5-12.0 mcg/dL
Optimal goal: 8-10 mcg/dL*

Total T4 is considered to reflect the body's storage form of thyroid hormone, both free and bound to protein. The body needs an adequate amount of T4 in order to convert to T3, which is the active thyroid hormone. Most of the thyroid hormone produced by the body is in the form of T4, while a small percentage of T3 is produced. T4, however, is mostly inactive while T3 is the active hormone. Very little of T3 is actually produced by the thyroid gland; the liver is responsible for a lot of the conversion. Mineral deficiencies, digestive challenges, and adrenal fatigue are among the factors that can inhibit the conversion. I have found that patients whose test results show difficulty converting T4 to T3 also have low selenium, chronic constipation, and/or high-stress lifestyles.[14, 16] (See Chapter 6 for more information about the adrenals and the thyroid.)

Free T4

Normal range: 0.8-1.8 ng/dL
Optimal goal: 1.3-1.8 ng/dL*

Free T4 is considered to be the storage form of thyroid circulating in the blood, unbound to protein. If this level is low, it may be an indicator that a T4-specific thyroid medication such as Synthroid or a nutritional supplement may be beneficial. This goal range is especially important if low thyroid symptoms exist, such as headaches, cold hands and feet, and/or hair loss.[17]

Free T3

Normal range: 2.3-4.2 ng/mL
Optimal goal: 3.1-4.2 ng/mL*

Free T3 is considered to be the active thyroid hormone circulating in the blood, unbound to protein. This level is more directly tied to low energy, weight gain, low moods, and headaches. T3 co-localizes with serotonin receptors in the brain. Serotonin is one of the mood-stabilizing, pain-relieving neurotransmitters, so this may suggest the importance of maintaining an optimal Free T3. If the Free T3 level is too low, it is often important to consider adrenal issues. I have observed that adrenal fatigue is often found in individuals with low T3 levels. It is extremely important to always support the adrenals with nutritional supplements or herbs while taking a thyroid hormone medication. This goal range is essential for anyone who suffers with any neurological condition.[18-20]

Reverse T3

Normal range: 11-32 ng/dL
Optimal goal: 11-20 ng/dL*

Reverse T3 (rT3) is considered to be the storage form of T3. As previously mentioned, stress inhibits the body's ability to convert T4 to T3. Under duress, the body chooses to manufacture cortisol instead of T3 since they are both very stimulating to the nervous system. It's the body's way of maintaining harmony. Unfortunately, cortisol suppresses the thyroid and low thyroid symptoms may appear during this time. When Reverse T3 is within the goal range, it is a marker that you are appropriately utilizing the T3 that is present in your body. If Reverse T3 is high, it signals that your body is storing T3 rather than using it. The body is unable to function optimally in terms of energy, moods, and pain cycling.[21]

Thyroid Peroxidase Antibodies

Normal range: <35 IU/mL
Optimal goal: <35 IU/mL*

This enzyme is important in the production of thyroid hormones. If this level is high, your immune system is overly active, which is often seen in imbalanced Pitta dosha types. Instead of creating antibodies to protect you, the body produces antibodies to attack your natural enzyme system in the thyroid, which leads to inflammation of the gland and possible dysfunction in hormone production.[22] If elevated, certain protocols have to be put in place to reduce the production. These protocols include avoiding gluten, removing mercury fillings, reducing mercury consumption, and healing your digestive system, along with lifestyle measures to reduce your Pitta fire.

Your Hormones and Migraines

An essential component of my protocol to modulate and control migraine headaches is to make sure that the body's hormones are in balance. The following is an explanation of the optimal range for hormones.

Cholesterol

Normal range: 125-200 mg/dL
Optimal goal: 180-200 mg/dL*

Cholesterol is a hormone with a bad reputation, but it's not so bad when it's in balance. We actually need cholesterol — it's the mother of all hormones. Cholesterol is responsible for synthesizing the precursor hormone pregnenolone, which is responsible for many essential functions of the body. Pregnenolone, in turn, is the precursor for other important hormones, including DHEA, cortisol, estrogen, testosterone, and progesterone.[23] Having high cholesterol could be a sign of inflammation in the body. When the body is in need of hormones such as cortisol to shield it from inflammation (as occurs in migraines), the body tends to produce more cholesterol to compensate *(Figure 4)*.

The Steroid Hormone Pathway:
It All Begins With Cholesterol (Figure 4)[24]

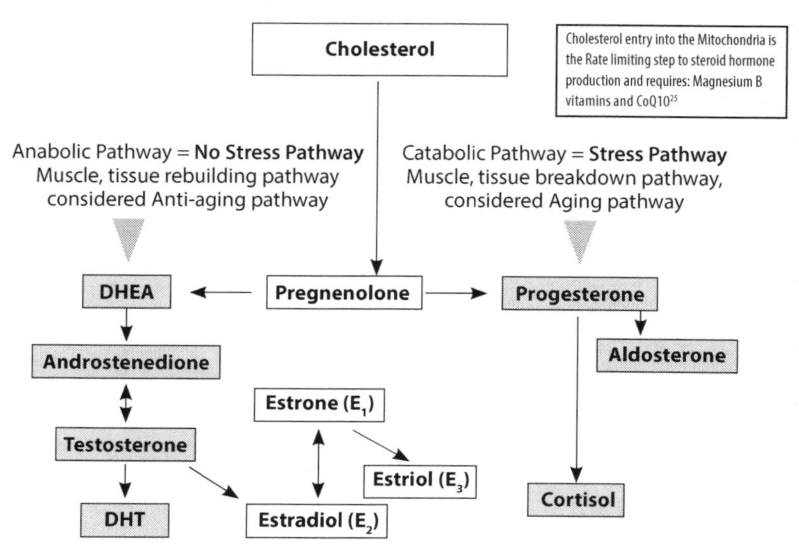

Cholesterol, after converting to pregnenolone, has a choice to enter the anabolic pathway or the catabolic pathway based on the needs of each of our cells and our body's requirements at that moment.

Which pathway does your body/mind choose each day, the anti-aging "no stress" pathway or the aging "stress" pathway?

DHEA

Normal range: <145 mcg/dL
Optimal goal: 80-120 mcg/dL*

DHEA is a hormone produced in the adrenal glands and sex organs. DHEA is essential for vitality and for rebounding from stress and trauma. DHEA is often reported in laboratory tests in ratio to cortisol. This ratio is important because it indicates the patient's adrenal health and stress level. Depletion of DHEA is a marker of long-term stress.

Optimal range varies with each individual, based on genetics and dosha type. DHEA can help the immune system and is often needed to replenish low testosterone levels, which can help migraines. Since it buffers cortisol, it can help manage stress. Generally, we should maintain a very specific ratio of DHEA to cortisol. In our stressed nation, DHEA levels often run quite low in our patient population.[26]

Progesterone

Normal range: 2.6-21.5 ng/mL luteal phase

Progesterone has a calming effect on the nervous system since it binds with GABA receptors (chemical messengers widely distributed throughout the brain).[27] I have found that the majority of female patients in my practice with migraine also have low progesterone levels during their menstrual cycle (luteal phase). In our center, we collected saliva samples from 90 women and found that 87% were low progesterone.

Based on clinical symptoms, Vata dosha types — with an anxious mind and difficulty falling asleep — may benefit from the calming effect of progesterone. In addition, irritable Pitta dosha types may find themselves feeling more relaxed from taking this hormone, especially if they have menstrual migraines. Saliva results and doshic state are used to assess dosing.

Estradiol

Normal range: 56-214 pg/mL luteal phase

Did you know that we manufacture three types of estrogens? Estrogen hormones in the body circulate as estriol, estradiol, and estrone. Prior to menopause, the estrogen most prominent is estradiol. This is also the estrogen that has the strongest effect on the brain.[28,29]

Estrogen is essential for developing a strong memory and enhanced thought processes. However, too much estrogen can create an overly excitable nervous system. It is also very important to consider the ratio of estradiol to progesterone. Too much estradiol in relation to progesterone can lead to estrogen dominance, a condition that is at the root of accelerated aging, allergies, gallbladder issues, fibrocystic growths, and some cancers.[30]

Based on clinical symptoms and dosha type, estradiol can be helpful for migraine patients, especially if given with estriol. Estrogens in any form should always be given with progesterone, whether the uterus is present or not.[31] A compounding pharmacist can create a topical, combination cream form of these estrogens, based on matching clinical symptoms to salivary levels.[32]

Ferritin

Normal range: 10-232 ng/mL
Optimal goal: 70-100 ng/mL*

Ferritin is the measure of the body's stored iron. In many neurological conditions, especially migraine and restless leg syndrome, low ferritin can worsen the condition. Iron carries oxygen to cells; without oxygen, the cells often become excitable. Ferritin also enhances thyroid hormone production. It is very important to check this level and treat it if the thyroid is also found to be low, or if the patient complains of low thyroid symptoms such as fatigue, weight gain, cold hands and feet, constipation, and/or brain fog.

Often a low ferritin level is a sign of a weak digestive system as the body may not be breaking down proteins well. Addressing digestion is also important if this level is low. With low ferritin levels, there is a risk of poor oxygenation of the nervous system and low thyroid function, which can increase migraines if not corrected.[33]

Vitamin B12

Normal range: 200-1100 pg/mL
Optimal goal: 600-900 pg/mL*

Vitamin B12 is needed for adrenal-cortisol production. B12 can also help individuals with low energy, poor memory, and numbness or tingling in their extremities. The best source of this vitamin is medical-grade supplements or B12 injections. The beauty of B12 is that it is a water-soluble vitamin. That means you can take higher dosages to improve symptoms, because toxicity is rare.[34]

Additional Tests That Can Make the Difference

Food Sensitivity Testing

Food sensitivity is discussed in detail in Chapter 5. Keep in mind that eliminating a single food such as wheat can radically change your health for the better. Please do this only under the guidance of a trained professional, as simply eliminating a food without actively repairing the digestive system may lead to problems down the road.

Adrenal and Hormone Saliva Testing

This test, often conducted by submitting saliva samples taken at home throughout the course of the day, provides an assessment of the body's daily cortisol release. The highest amount of cortisol is usually released by the body in the morning. The levels decrease at noon and again at 3 p.m., and are very low around bedtime. This test reveals the various stages of adrenal function that could be impacting your well-being (discussed in detail in Chapter 6). Also, measuring salivary hormones during the menstrual cycle provides a more accurate glimpse of the hormonal balance in women.

Celiac and *H. pylori* Testing

In certain cases, this test can be very helpful in evaluating digestive health. Celiac disease is an extreme allergy to gluten and wheat. If it is untreated, celiac can lead to autoimmune disease, digestive issues, growth retardation, and neurological sequelae (a disorder of the nervous system resulting from another disease).[35]

H. pylori is a bacterial infection in the stomach that usually begins in childhood. It damages the protective mucous lining of the stomach and small intestine and hinders your body's ability to absorb nutrients.

Taking the Next Step

Based on your clinical picture, some or all of these tests may be recommended. In truth, most clinicians are able to get a picture of which areas need support without the need to test. We often prefer to begin supplement protocols in hope of balancing the system and relieving symptoms. If this does not occur, we would then consider testing in hope that we may find that the system is more imbalanced than we imagined. Remember that your clinical picture is far more valuable than a test result. Once the results show what conditions are present, dietary changes and nutritional supplements are the optimal forms of treatment to help restore your health and vitality. You'll learn more about these forms of treatment in Part III.

Armed with these clues surrounding your body's biochemistry, you're one step closer to solving the mystery of your pain and discomfort. Let's unravel another clue, the impact of food sensitivities on your health, in the next chapter.

---

* *These ranges were based on discussions and information received at the Institute of Functional Medicine Course on Hormone Balancing 2012.*

CHAPTER 5
The Gut-Brain Link

"Let food be thy medicine, thy medicine be thy food."
Hippocrates

There are moments in our lives that forever change us. I had been struggling to help one of my dear patients, Eva, who had been suffering from daily headaches along with migraines. Eva was only 13 years old when I first started seeing her. During her initial visit, we discussed the stress of school and challenges of adolescence, and I decided to place her on some natural daily supplements and give her an abortive medication to rid her severe attacks of pain when they came on. The headaches continued to progress, and thus we decided to add a stronger daily medication to her regimen, along with trigger point injections to control her pain. Although her headaches did improve in intensity and frequency, we still had not been able to figure out why she suffered with so many headaches at such a young age. We discussed obtaining a Vitamin D level and doing food allergy testing in hopes of finding the cause of her pain.

On her own, Eva decided to go gluten-free. Within three months, Eva's headaches dramatically improved. She explained, "Before I went on a gluten-free diet, I suffered from severe migraines that would force me to lay in my dark, quiet bedroom for a couple of days a month, and I had mild to moderate headaches almost every day. When I changed my diet, the relief was instant; the migraines no longer lasted days and I was able to function while I had one. Thanks to a gluten-free diet, I now suffer from short migraines about once a month and I no longer have a daily headache."

After witnessing dramatic results in Eva, I began a quest to understand the link between digestion and the brain (the gut-brain link, *see Figure 3*) and the impact of food sensitivities or intolerances on neurological health.

Gut-Brain Link (Figure 3)

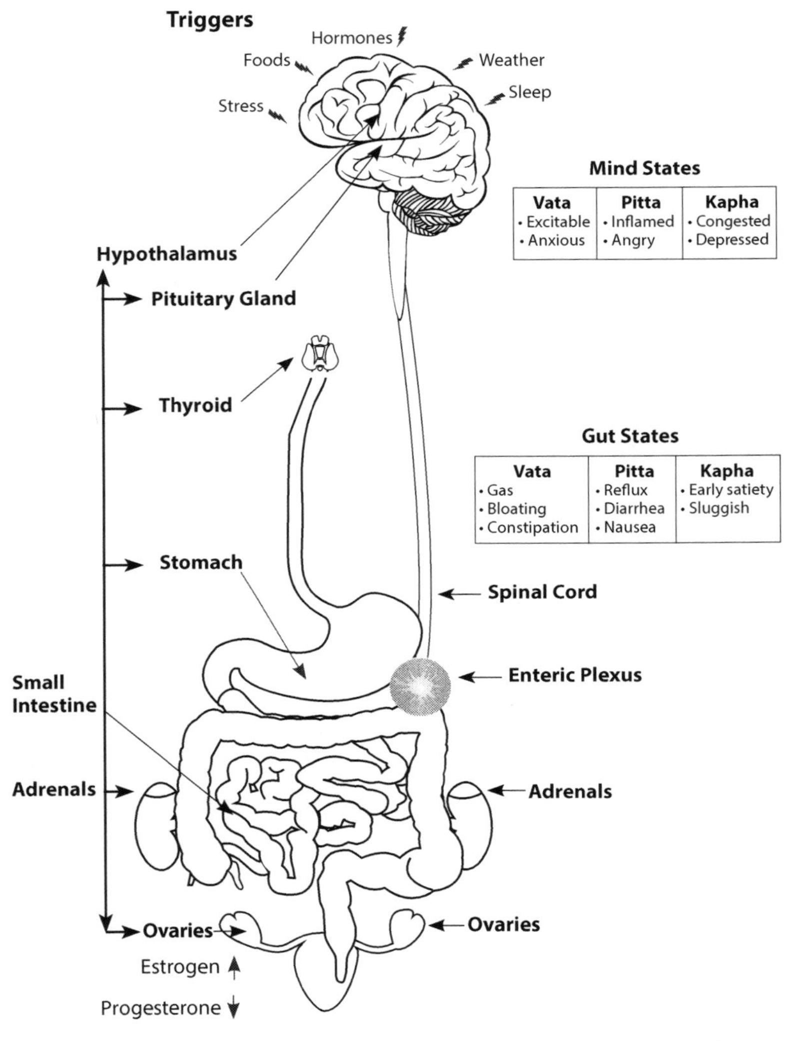

Mind States

Vata	Pitta	Kapha
• Excitable • Anxious	• Inflamed • Angry	• Congested • Depressed

Gut States

Vata	Pitta	Kapha
• Gas • Bloating • Constipation	• Reflux • Diarrhea • Nausea	• Early satiety • Sluggish

The key to understanding neurological symptoms, such as headaches, insomnia, mood issues and fatigue, is the realization that there is a strong link between the gut and brain. In addition, the nervous system is intimately connected to our adrenal system, ovaries and thyroid gland. When the brain becomes excitable, inflamed and/or congested, it often is a result of the adrenals, ovaries and thyroid system not being in optimal balance. Balancing these organs can strengthen the brain and improve brain function.

Sample Food Sensitivity Chart (Figure 5)

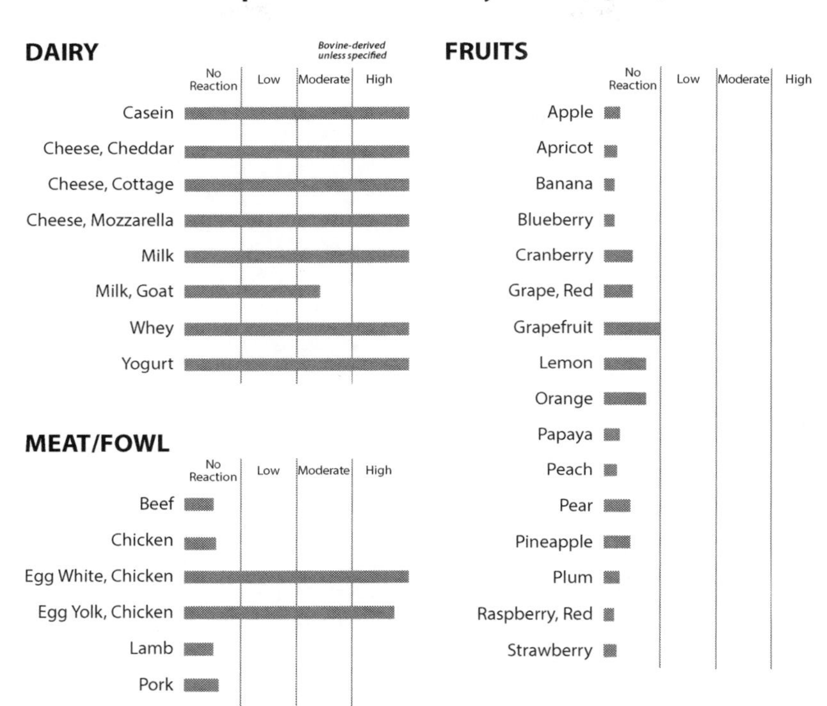

Sample Food Sensitivity Chart (Continued)

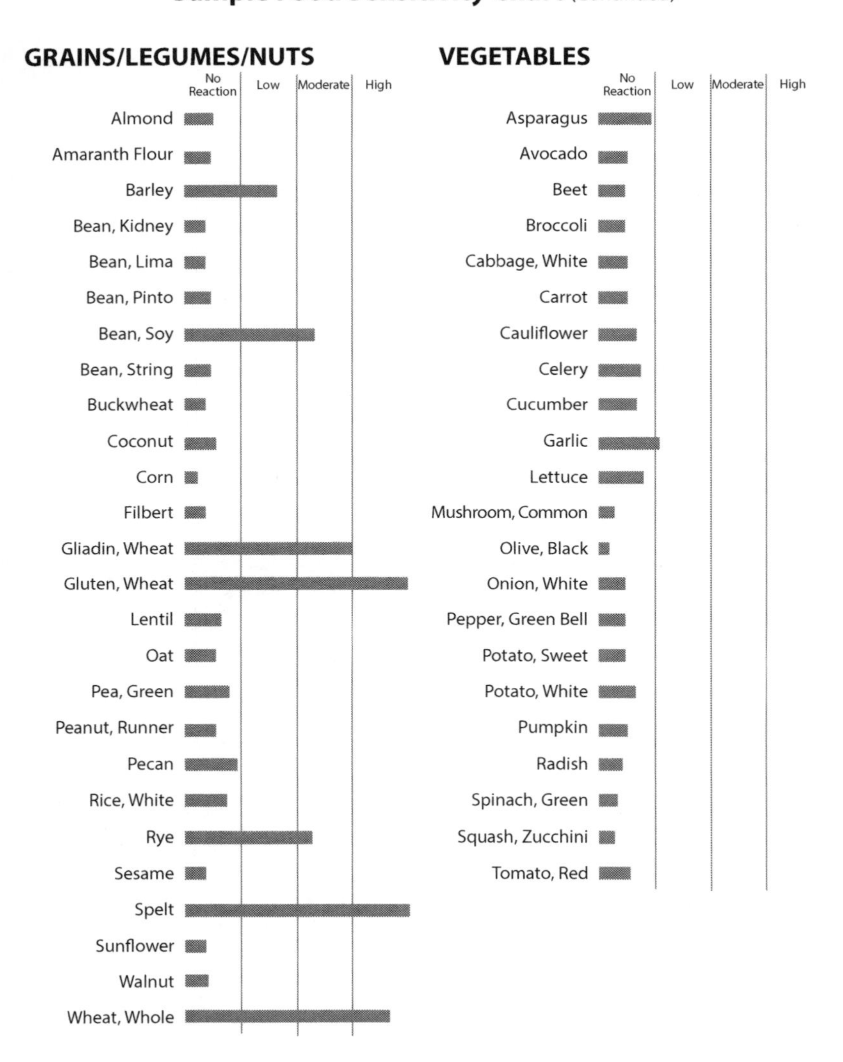

In this sample chart, items that are in the 'no reaction' area are of low risk in triggering a systemic reaction. Those in the 'moderate-to-high' reaction area are more likely to lead to inflammation in digestion and, thus, more systemic reactions.

In addition to reviewing many studies, I began testing patients in my own practice. Using food sensitivity blood testing that looks for IgG antibody responses, I tested 500 patients. The results were both startling and illuminating:

Food Group	Percentage of Patients Affected
Dairy	59% moderate to severe IgG response
Egg white and yolk	36% moderate to severe IgG response
Grains (including wheat)	47% moderate to severe IgG response

Keep in mind that it takes between 4 and 72 hours for the IgG antibody response to develop. For example, you could eat a piece of cheese today and not show any antibody response for three days. No wonder the foods I tested were often labeled "hidden food sensitivities." These sensitivities, also referred to as "food intolerances," can lead to a wide array of symptoms including (but not limited to) fatigue, low moods, difficulty focusing, pronounced digestive symptoms, and headaches.

Not long after I began testing my own patients for food sensitivities, my then five-year-old daughter began having headaches. The symptoms were troubling to me because, besides what I thought were the normal runny noses and ear infections that plagued young children, she had been a relatively healthy child and had met all of the growth and developmental milestones. Due to the incredible improvements my migraine patients experienced after food sensitivity testing followed by food elimination and digestive strengthening, I decided to have the tests administered to my daughter. To my surprise, the results showed a high sensitivity to dairy, eggs, and gluten.

Soon after my daughter began having headaches, my son would wake up from a sound sleep, crying in distress with an episode of vomiting. These episodes occurred nightly for about two months and were disturbing and disrupting for our entire family. Each night when this occurred I would wash his mouth and body while my husband changed the crib sheets. Upon discovering that my daughter had food sensitivities, I decided to have my son tested. The results showed that my son had extremely high intolerance to dairy and eggs. Guess what? I had been giving him a bottle of milk every night before bed. I never connected the dots between the milk and the vomiting, though looking back now it seems extremely obvious.

I was also troubled that his very intelligent pediatrician recommended a CT scan of the head (high resolution x-ray) and an upper GI test (to explore the esophagus, stomach, and small intestine) to determine the cause of the vomiting episodes. She never once asked what I fed him. I'm not being judgmental of her; she was a very caring and compassionate doctor. I know from personal experience that nutritional education is a very small fraction of traditional medical training. Nonetheless, I am relieved that I was able to get to the root cause of my son's vomiting so that he would not have to follow her recommendation of starting the medication Pepcid, an acid blocker, in an effort to treat what she diagnosed as "reflux." I feel blessed that I had the testing kits available in my office and had the skills and knowledge to interpret the results and implement digestive protocols for my children.

I immediately placed both of my children on a restricted diet and added probiotics, digestive enzymes, and vitamin D3. The headaches and vomiting ceased within a short time. After following the restricted food plan for a few months, I slowly re-introduced some of those foods to their diet. However, I limited the consumption to only a few times per week. I still continue the regimen of probiotics, digestive enzymes, and vitamin D3 to this day. I also added omega-3 essential fatty acids to continue to support their digestive systems.

It's important to note that when I increase my children's consumption of dairy and eggs, they both have a tendency to develop digestive issues and/or congestion. My daughter even gets fevers and earaches when she overconsumes these items. Looking back, given what I know now, I wonder if my daughter's repeated ear infections when she was a toddler were a manifestation of a "hidden intolerance" to the dairy, egg, or wheat products which I was feeding her daily because I believed these items were healthy. My perception of healthy eating is now quite different than at that time. Foods that create allergy are surely not healthy!

What Causes Food Sensitivities?

The seven most common food sensitivities are corn, eggs, dairy products, soy, cane sugar (including fructose, dextrose, and maltose), wheat, and yeast. Food intolerance or sensitivity can be due to one or more factors, such as:

The inability of your body to digest a certain food due to insufficiency in a digestive enzyme or stomach acid. An estimated 70 to 90% of people of Greek, Asian, and African descent are lactose intolerant because their bodies do not produce the enzyme lactase. For some, switching to lactose-free foods may not be a viable option. Lactose is a milk sugar. Manufacturers of lactose-free milks often substitute casein and whey for lactose, but they also are milk proteins. Many patients who are lactose intolerant also can't eat casein and whey.

An adverse reaction to products in foods such as preservatives or additives to enhance color and taste. Most processed foods today are overloaded with dyes (especially yellow dye #5) and preservatives, such as monosodium glutamate, most commonly known as MSG. There are more than 40 different ingredients that contain the chemical in MSG, processed-free glutamic acid. More information is available at www.truthinlabeling.org, which has a free list available for download. MSG-reaction triggers can also be caused by products containing rice syrup, brown rice syrup, milk powder, and most things labeled "enriched" or "low fat." Glutamate is an excitatory transmitter in the nervous system which may lead to symptoms of flushing, facial pressure, headache, and warmth. Sulfites are another common additive. They are often present in wine and dried fruits and are used to prevent mold.

Histamine content. Foods high in histamine are often responsible for many food intolerances. Symptoms of intolerance to these foods — ranging from sinus congestion to gas — can begin within minutes or days after ingesting them. Foods rich in histamine include aged cheeses; processed meats; red, white, or sparkling wine; beer; smoked fish; tuna and mackerel (especially if not refrigerated); and pineapple, mango, pears, raspberries, and kiwi. The natural food enzyme that breaks down histamine is known as Diamine Oxidase (DAO). This enzyme is responsible for reducing histamine levels that can lead to food intolerances. There have been many research studies about the connection between histamines and migraines. However, the study that has recently received the most recognition was one conducted by researchers in Spain:[36]

Researchers found that almost 90 percent of migraine sufferers were also deficient in the enzyme DAO, which is needed to help metabolize histamine during an allergic reaction. The researchers, based at International University of Catalonia, studied 137 subjects with episodic migraines. After administering oral DAO supplements to patients with each of their daily meals, fewer and shorter migraine attacks were reported. While there were no noted adverse effects, there also was no significant reduction in pain reported as a result of the enzyme migraine treatment.[37]

The ancient science of Ayurveda may have more accurate and applicable insights on the function of the human body than was previously understood, despite the lack of technological support to back its findings. One of the Ayurvedic recommendations is to avoid packaged or leftover foods, as they are considered to impair health long term. The more aged or ripened the food, the higher the histamine content. This Ayurvedic principle may now be better understood based on the science presented above regarding deficient enzyme activity needed to metabolize histamine.

Are Sensitivity Tests Effective?

Although there is debate in the conventional medical community about the efficacy of blood testing for food allergies and sensitivities, my experience has taught me that they are both essential and invaluable in the treatment of migraines and the effort to help my patients improve the quality of their overall health. These blood tests measure your immune system's response to particular foods by checking the amount of allergy-type antibodies in your bloodstream, known as Immunoglobulin E (IgE) antibodies, and/or the amount of Immunoglobulin G (IgG) mediated immune responses.

IgE (or Immunoglobulin E) allergies are immediate reactions to what the body perceives as a foreign substance that has either been eaten or inhaled. IgE allergy symptoms include difficulty breathing and/or swelling and can range from mild to life-threatening, such as anaphylactic shock. Food allergies impact multiple systems of the body. Other symptoms of allergies include vomiting, stomach cramps, hives, itchy eyes or nose, sneezing, nasal congestion, and throat tightness.

Food sensitivity is an adverse reaction to a food with no antigen-antibody response in the blood. The Immunoglobulin G (IgG) test reveals food sensitivities that have become much more prevalent. I believe the increase in food sensitivities is due to an overconsumption of processed foods, wheat and dairy products, and refined sugars, along with chronic dehydration. Coupled with poor eating habits, such as eating at the wrong times or simply not chewing your food enough before swallowing, food sensitivities have become chronic, underlying causes of migraines. Symptoms of food sensitivities include headache, nausea, hyperactivity, and autoimmune disease. Some people experience extreme fatigue or bloating after eating a food to which they are sensitive. They can also experience mood changes. People with chronic food sensitivities also have dark circles or puffiness under the eyes. A reaction can occur hours or even days after the offending food has been ingested.

When the digestive lining is perfectly intact with adequate Secretory IgA (sIgA) levels, these types of reactions are not able to occur. The sIgA level is an important indicator of digestive-immune function. Low levels can lead to recurrent infections and food intolerances. Anyone with a high food sensitivity score likely has low sIgA levels and a "leaky gut."

Leaky Gut Syndrome

Much debate exists between the conventional and integrative medical communities concerning the origin of food allergies. Since the traditional American diet is heavily weighted toward processed foods, an abundance of chemical additives (including salt and sugar) are believed to be potential triggers. When the body is unable to naturally create the enzymes or digestive acids necessary to process the "protein portion" of that food, it sets off a cascade of challenges in the body. This is referred to as "leaky gut syndrome." Leaky gut syndrome is not generally recognized by conventional medicine, and there are limited treatment protocols using pharmaceutical drugs. However, the alternative medical community has been openly addressing and advocating treatment for this syndrome for more than 20 years.

According to Andrew Weil, MD, author and alternative medicine pioneer, there is mounting evidence that "leaky gut" is a real condition that affects the lining of the intestines. Dr. Weil notes that "leaky gut syndrome (also called increased intestinal permeability) is the result of damage to the intestinal lining, making it less able to protect the internal environment as well as to filter needed nutrients and other biological substances. As a consequence, some bacteria and their toxins, incompletely digested proteins and fats, and waste which are not normally absorbed may 'leak' out of the intestines into the blood stream."[38]

Alternative medical professionals believe that leaky gut syndrome can trigger an autoimmune reaction, which can lead to gastrointestinal problems such as abdominal bloating, excessive gas and cramps, fatigue, food sensitivities, joint pain, skin rashes, and autoimmunity. The cause of this syndrome may be chronic inflammation, food sensitivity, damage from taking large amounts of nonsteroidal anti-inflammatory drugs (NSAIDs), cytotoxic drugs and radiation, certain antibiotics, excessive alcohol consumption, or compromised immunity. Leaky gut can then potentially lead to the development of inflammation elsewhere in the body.

As you can see, digestive health is essential to maintaining total system health. If the immune system breaks down in the gut, this can lead to inflammation in other parts of the body such as muscles, joints, and organs, including the brain. That's why it's important for anyone with neurological symptoms, especially headaches, to take a closer look at the health of their digestive system.

Candida albicans: An Opportunistic, Health-Wrecking Fungus

Another potential source of food intolerance and/or allergies is an overgrowth of *Candida albicans,* which is an opportunistic fungus, or form of yeast, found in the mouth and intestines. Everyone has *Candida albicans.* However, it becomes a problem when chronic stress, a diet rich in carbohydrates and sugar, use of oral contraceptives, alcohol or drug abuse, and/or the extended use of antibiotics or other pharmaceutical drugs can cause it to spread uncontrolled. Out-of-control *Candida albicans* weakens the intestinal wall, eventually releasing its toxic byproducts throughout the body. These toxic byproducts cause damage to your body tissues and organs, wreaking havoc on your immune system.

The major waste product of yeast cell activity is a poisonous toxin called Acetaldehyde, which promotes free radical activity in the body.

Acetaldehyde is also converted by the liver into ethanol (drinking alcohol), leaving some people feeling drunk or hung-over with debilitating fatigue. Many sufferers of *Candida albicans* (also referred to as Candidiasis) are undiagnosed by their conventional medical doctors who treat the effects of Candidiasis, such as oral thrush or vaginal infections, and not the root cause.

Excessive craving of sweets is another symptom of Candidiasis, which leads to further candida growth and more sweet cravings. It's a vicious cycle of overgrowth and cravings. The central nervous system is extremely vulnerable to Candidiasis — depression, brain fog, headaches, and chronic fatigue are symptoms most notably associated with Candidiasis.

Taking the Next Step

In the next chapter, you'll learn about another underlying factor that may be contributing to the mystery of your health challenges and how you can use this clue to restore your vitality.

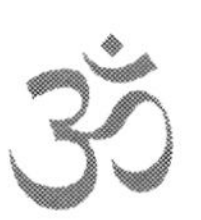

CHAPTER 6
Adrenal Fatigue: A Hidden Pervasive Syndrome

"Nature does not hurry, yet everything is accomplished."
Lao Tzu

At the risk of losing their lives, my parents fled Africa during the time of the Ugandan exodus of Southeast Asians and brought my siblings and me to the United States in search of a better life. As my family pursued the American dream, my mother never wanted us to take our lives for granted. From a very young age she insisted that we work very hard to succeed, which required focus, determination, and effort. This was not a choice; we had to prove to my parents that their risks and the journey they took to provide us with safety and opportunity were worth the sacrifice.

Today, the value of hard work is not limited to my experience or to the experiences of other immigrants. It's a pervasive part of the values of any individual or group of people who want to get ahead. Consequently, we judge ourselves as unproductive unless we're busy or constantly making efforts toward our goals. Of course, our motivation to succeed is often fueled by tangible rewards such as a job promotion, more income, a bigger home, a nicer car, a better wardrobe, or successful children. Never mind that we rarely take the time to enjoy the fruits of our labor because we're all too busy keeping up with the activities that make us even more tired.

Here is an interesting fact: the average American employee receives two weeks of paid vacation per year. Compare this to our European counterparts, who generally receive and take six weeks of paid vacation per year! It is no surprise that many of us do not take the vacation time we have earned. The downside to our culture's socially-accepted workaholic or "stay busy" syndrome is that we do not know how to let go and relax.

During the 2012 presidential campaign, Mitt Romney warned that European-style benefits would "poison the very spirit of America." However, I had a totally different experience during the month I spent in Spain between my first and second year of medical school. As a result, I developed a deeper understanding of why Europeans don't have the same health problems or challenges with their healthcare system as we do in the U.S.

During that month, I arrived at the hospital each morning at 9 a.m., ready to work. My mentor-physician smiled and greeted me daily by saying, "You Americans work so hard! Just enjoy!" He then encouraged me to sip a cup of coffee (not guzzle as we do here) and socialize until 10 a.m. We worked until noon, then left to eat a large lunch. Lunch was followed by a siesta. We returned to the hospital after the siesta and worked until 5 p.m. I remember that the waiting room was still filled with patients as we departed work for the day. However, instead of staying late, my mentor-physician said, "They can wait until tomorrow to be seen. There's nothing urgent going on with any of them."

These physicians treated their patients well. However, they did not sacrifice their personal time by squeezing into one day all the patients waiting to be seen. I was also amazed to see that the medical staff never skipped lunch in order to see more patients. When it was 5 p.m. and time to go home and unwind, they listened to the call of Mother Nature and ended their work day. They did not push their limits or stress their systems by overworking.

Looking back, I remember how happy and friendly the physicians and staff were at all times. Very few of them were moody. This was quite a contrast to the physicians I had met or studied with in the United States.

Studying in Spain was an eye-opening experience for me, teaching me important lessons in attending to my needs as a provider (not that I would ever leave a waiting room filled with patients and expect them to return the next day!). At the time, I was a highly-motivated, highly-stressed, hard-driving perfectionist — characteristics I deemed necessary to becoming a good physician. Although I went to Spain to learn more about patient care, the real lesson of my experience was the importance of self-care by creating balance among work, rest, and play. That balance is necessary in order to have the energy and life force to take care of others.

We surely have a lot to learn from our European counterparts. Providing excellent care for patients also involves teaching them how to observe and follow the patterns of nature, to manage stress, and to nurture themselves. To teach them well, it's important that the physician or healthcare provider first model that behavior.

The Potentially Fatal Curse of Stress

The word "stress" is a shortened version of the term "distress." According to the *Oxford Dictionary*, it evolves from Latin and means "to draw or pull apart." Today, stress is an epidemic that leaves us feeling *ripped* apart. I believe it is the root cause of our nation's healthcare crisis, impacting men, women, and children. Unfortunately, many of us have no idea how to function without stress! I believe that's because we don't understand its potential, long-lasting, and debilitating effects.

The late Dr. Hans Selye was a pioneering neuro-endocrinologist from Hungary who has been dubbed "the father of stress research." He coined the term "general adaptation syndrome" to describe the three phases of stress (alarm, resistance, and exhaustion) and the impact it has on the body.[39] After many years of research, Dr. Selye concluded that stress is a major cause of disease because chronic stress causes long-term chemical changes in the body.[40]

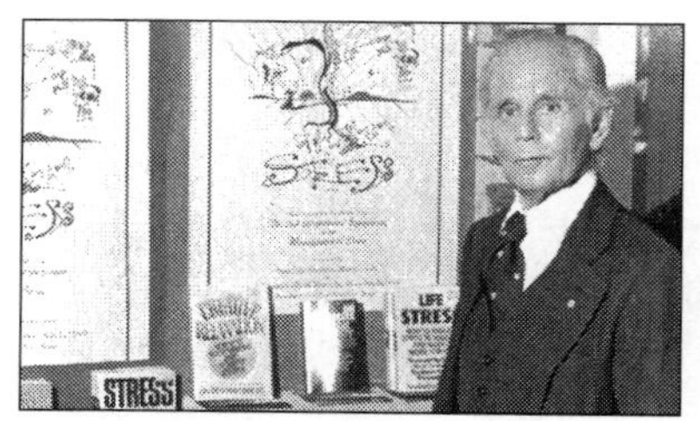

Management Division of Records and Archives, University of Montreal. Hans Selye Collection (p0359). 1FP07740 . Hans Selye in front of his books on stress.

Chronic stress has been found to cause damage to the nerve cells in tissues and organs, leading to an inability to process information, impaired memory, and a tendency toward anxiety and/or depression. When I began to probe the neurological impacts of stress on the brain, I learned that optimal nervous system function requires nourishment with an appropriate amount of cortisol, DHEA, estrogen, progesterone, and thyroid hormone, along with other hormones. These hormones, when appropriately released in the correct amounts and ratios, have a tremendous ability to impact the nervous system from becoming excitable and inflamed during stressful situations. An intact circadian rhythm that follows the rhythm of nature is key to maintaining a healthy balance between the brain and body.

The Flight or Fight Response

When you have a stressful experience, your body provides instant protection by giving you a sudden jolt of hormones. In an instant, you are equipped with the energy to handle the situation. Health challenges begin to manifest in the body when you repeatedly experience stress with little or no time to recover (think of a blaring fire alarm that you can never turn off). When stress occurs, we either stay in the midst of stress and try to manage the stress to our best ability, or we run from it. This is from where the phrase "flight or fight" was derived. If you choose to stay with the stressor, over the course of time your body loses its ability to handle the stress because the energy supply needed to adapt is totally depleted. This is often referred to by Western medical doctors as overload, burnout, adrenal fatigue, maladaptation, or dysfunction. This is when your adrenal glands (which produce stress hormones) turn on and stay on, leading to a point when your adrenals eventually shut down. This can continue until the body becomes depleted. It is this phase — exhaustion — that is the most hazardous to your health. Because your ability to manage stress is critical to your overall well-being, let's discuss how this happens in greater detail.

The hypothalamus is the brain's central processing gland, organizing and controlling the flow of information into and out of the brain and regulating the entire body. I like to think of the hypothalamus as the "mom," or central director of the body. Whenever the body is triggered by events such as stress, weather changes, hormonal fluctuations, or a particular food that has been ingested, the hypothalamus acknowledges that stressor and communicates with the rest of the body in an attempt to maintain harmony — "mom" wants to keep the peace. The hypothalamus warns the brain stem of the stressor and the brain stem attempts to recruit serotonin from the gut in order to calm the brain. However, if the digestive system is not in harmony, the gut is unable to manufacture enough serotonin, causing the brain stem to become undernourished and excitable. In this stage you may experience a tension headache, and if the brain can not be quieted at this stage, blood vessels become swollen and the brain becomes inflamed.

At this point, the hypothalamus is now communicating with the pituitary gland, which is also located in the brain *(See Figure 3)*. Together, these two glands relay information about the state of the body to the adrenals. The adrenal glands are your body's primary "stress absorbers," much like the shock absorbers on your car. Located on top of your kidneys, these walnut-sized organs produce several hormones necessary for responding to life — both good and challenging times. These hormones include norepinephrine, cortisol, and DHEA (discussed in detail later in this chapter). Cortisol works as an anti-inflammatory to block the inflamed brain, so your body will produce a lot of cortisol to attempt to break migraine pain *(See Figures 6 and 7)*. But when you're under chronic stress or chronic inflammation — be it from migraine, mood disorders, or foot pain — the adrenals become fatigued. Eventually the adrenals become overtaxed, cortisol and other hormone production drops, and the hypothalamus becomes desensitized — "mom" takes a back seat and gives up *(See Figure 8)*.

When the adrenals are turned on too intensely for too long, they simply cannot keep up with the constant and chronic production of hormones and neurotransmitters. Generally, epinephrine levels drop with cortisol and then norepinephrine levels drop, which leads to many common complaints such as memory problems and morning fatigue *(See Figure 8)*. Headaches and muscle and joint pain can ensue at this stage. When the adrenals are finally overburdened and unable to manufacture any hormones or neurotransmitters, a multitude of symptoms may occur, including difficulty dragging yourself out of bed, sweet cravings, recurrent infections, depression, and headaches.

In addition, when the adrenals are activated and they release high amounts of cortisol and norepinephrine, the thyroid gland is signaled to slow down. During times of stress, the body gives the thyroid a break and lets it relax. However, the body needs an active thyroid hormone (T3) to provide energy, suppress headaches, stabilize moods, and modulate weight. Living life out of harmony with your nature automatically stresses your adrenal system, thus possibly impairing thyroid function.

Hormones Produced by the Adrenal Glands

The hormones produced by the adrenal glands include norepinephrine, cortisol, and DHEA. Each of these hormones has a specific responsibility.

Norepinephrine (also called noradrenaline) and Epinephrine (also called adrenaline)

These are commonly thought of as the "flight or fight" hormones. The adrenals release these hormones when you feel as if you are in a threatening situation. When norepinephrine and epinephrine are simultaneously released, blood rushes to your heart, the pupils of your eyes enlarge, and you can develop inordinate muscular strength. Your tolerance for pain increases. Picture a man or woman suddenly being able to lift a car off of an injured person or suddenly being able to run fast to get out of harm's way.

I studied this neurotransmitter during functional medicine training, and I learned that when it is released from the locus coeruleus of the brain it has the effect of suppressing neuroinflammation. Common acetaminophen (Tylenol) also seems to have an effect on increasing norepinephrine levels in the brain. This may explain its effect on pain and why it is added to the list of many helpful, short-acting, abortive medications for headaches.

Cortisol

Cortisol helps the body resist the stressful effects of infection, trauma, and temperature extremes. Ideally, cortisol is only released when the body needs it, rather than continuously in response to chronic stress. When cortisol levels are too high, the impact can be devastating: potential loss of bone density, muscle wasting, kidney damage, increased blood sugar levels, weight gain, and greater vulnerability to bacteria, viruses, fungi, yeasts, allergies, parasites, and even cancer.

Dehydroepiandrosterone (DHEA)

DHEA is an androgen (hormone) produced by both the adrenal glands and the sex organs. DHEA neutralizes the impact that cortisol has on the immune system and is essential for vitality. In addition to helping you rebound from stress and trauma, DHEA also helps increase focus and maintain normal sleep patterns.

Adrenal Fatigue and Headache Medication

The adrenal glands manufacture neurotransmitters and steroid hormones, the most recognized of which is cortisol. Steroid medications such as prednisone are a stronger version of your own natural cortisol. When the adrenals cannot produce enough of these hormones, doctors recommend you take them in pill form. Steroid medications are one of the most common classes of pharmaceutical drugs prescribed to break a prolonged cycle of headaches. However, these drugs can actually create more issues with the adrenals and, if overused, they can worsen adrenal fatigue.[41]

In my early years of treating patients suffering with migraines, I was dismayed by the dizzying assortment of medications that I needed to prescribe to control pain — preventatives such as blood pressure medications, antidepressants, and seizure medications to decrease the number of headaches. I would euphemistically rename them "blood vessel regulating," "neurotransmitter balancing," and "neuromodulator" medications in hopes that these drugs were actually providing some sort of balance to an imbalanced system. I even started prescribing long-acting narcotic medications to quiet the pain when patients didn't respond to the initial medications.

However, after a couple of years, I felt as if I was defying the Hippocratic Oath taken during my medical school commencement ceremony, which encouraged us to be healers and to first "do no harm." I wanted to be a healer. I believed the role of the healer was to seek the root cause of the disease so that patients could achieve mind and body balance. Were the medications I prescribed allowing that process to occur? More importantly, was I doing any harm to the system by prescribing these medications?

I was most concerned about the risks associated with prescribing strong medications, often in combination, to quiet severe attacks, especially when the long-term effects of the medications were unknown. For example, there is data that suggests nutrient depletion is just one side effect of the long-term use of serotonin re-uptake inhibitors such as Prozac, and anti-seizure medications such as Topamax.[42] Consequently, I increased my efforts to find other ways to manage patients' headache pain.

Normal HPA Stress Response (Figure 6)

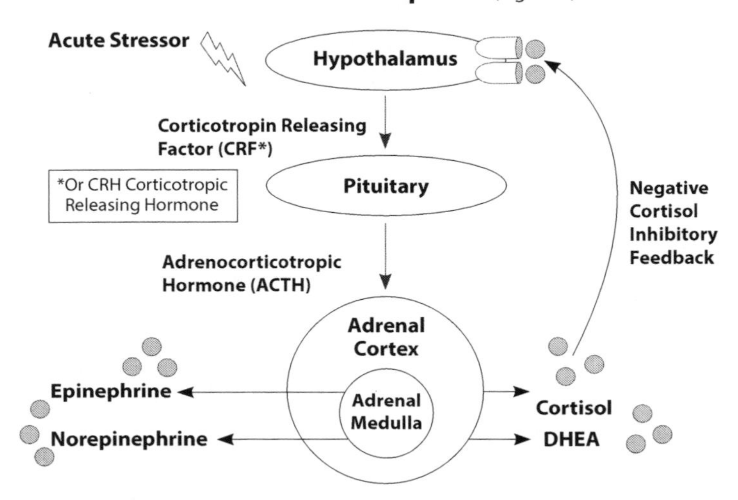

Under normal circumstances, an acute stressor (allergic food, weather shift, migraine attack) will lead to an adrenal release of cortisol, in hopes of relieving the stressor. Once the stress has passed, cortisol inhibits the hypothalamus and turns off the response.

Common Cortisol Ranges — Baseline/Normal (Figure 6A)

"Calm, healthy, energetic"

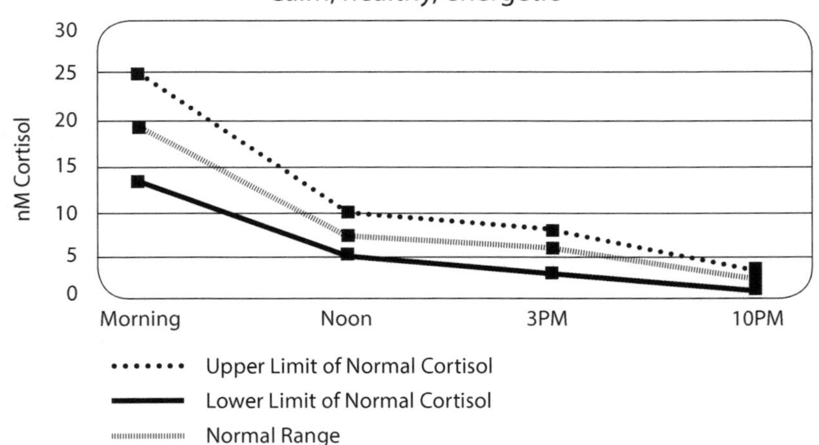

Normal Stress Response: During the day, we wake up and produce the highest amount of cortisol, which should fall between the upper and lower limit of normal. The cortisol production is reduced at lunchtime and then is very low at bedtime to allow for us to fall asleep. This was measured in our clinic by having patients collect saliva samples in the morning, noon, afternoon and bedtime, and then testing it for cortisol and other hormones.

Early Chronic HPA Stress Response (Figure 7)

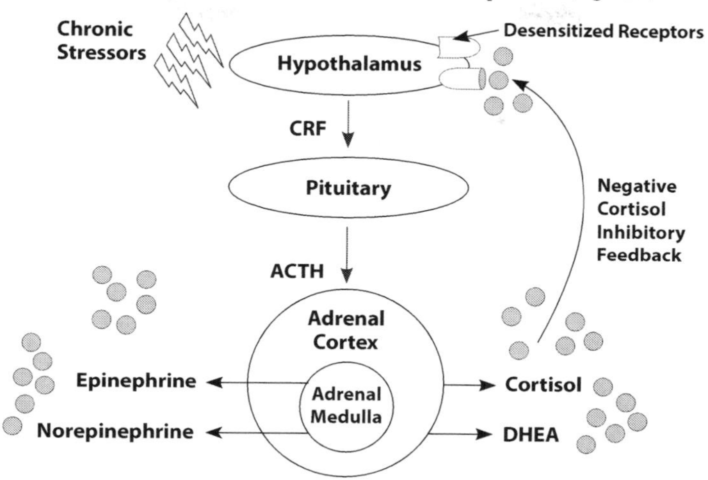

Stage 1: Alarm Stage — Nearly all cortisol levels at every time point tested are too high. During this time, we find individuals have an increased desire for sugar and caffeine to help maintain this driven state. During this stage, the individual is "on" and the cortisol findings are above the upper limit of a normal adrenal output.

Common Cortisol Ranges — Alarm Phase (Figure 7A)

"Stressed, wired, excitable"

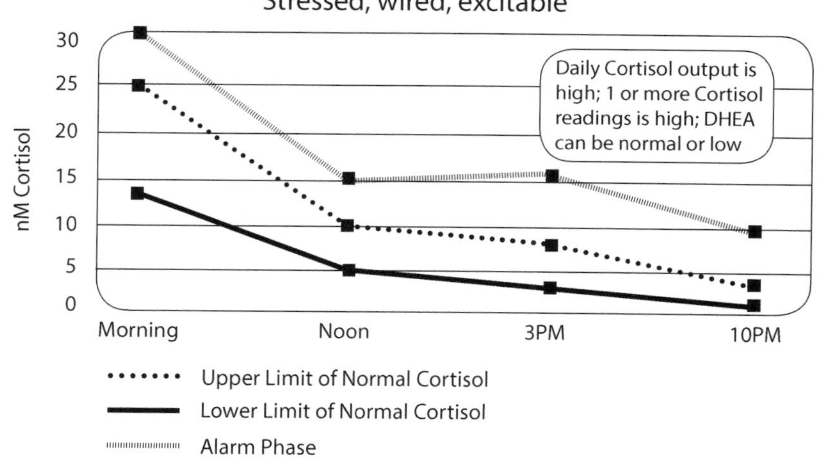

During this stage, the adrenals, due to input from the hypothalamus signaling chronic stress, release high levels of cortisol, along with the other adrenal hormones to help the mind and body handle the stress.

Mid-Stage Chronic HPA Stress Response (Figure 8)

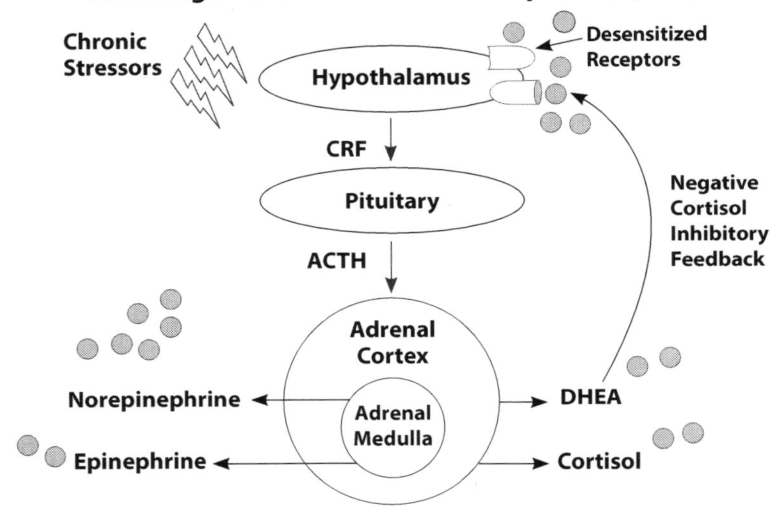

Stage 2: Resistance Stage — Most levels are low, though some may remain in range or high at night only. Thyroid and blood sugar disruption ensues, weight gain continues, and depression is common. The patient cannot function without sugar, caffeine, or medications such as a stimulant. The HPA axis begins to shut down.

Common Cortisol Ranges — Resistance Phase (Figure 8A)

"Fatigued in the morning, difficulty sleeping at night"

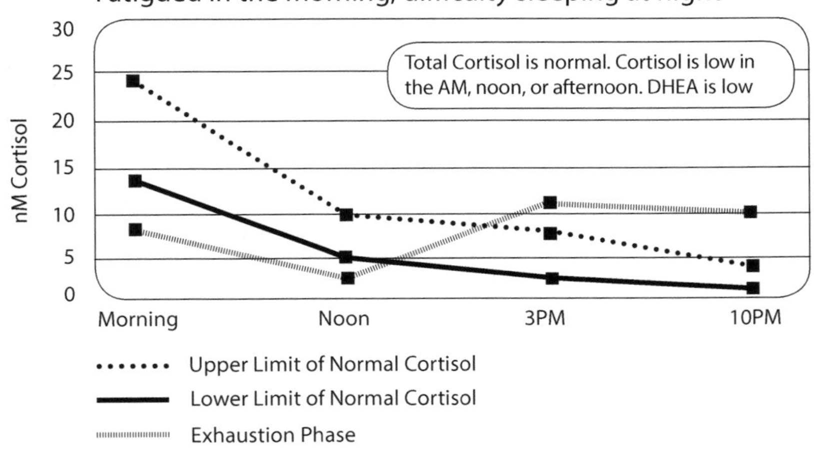

During this stage, since the adrenals have been "on" for too long, the adrenals start to fatigue, thus releasing less epinephrine and cortisol. Since it seems that the adrenals will not turn off soon, the hypothalamus starts to become desensitized to the ongoing stress response.

Late Stage Chronic HPA Stress Response (Figure 9)

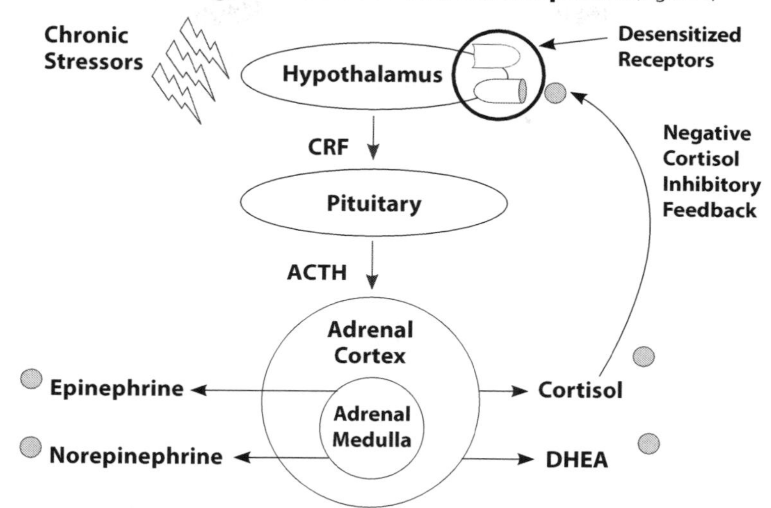

Stage 3: Exhaustion Stage — Nearly all levels are low as the HPA axis continues to shut down. Cardiovascular problems can occur at this stage. There is very little hormone reserve functioning; thus, dependency on external stimulants is the norm. Chronic pain is often present, along with chronic migraines. At this stage, not only are the adrenals weakened, but the hormone status is depleted, leaving the brain and body vulnerable and without protection.

Common Cortisol Ranges — Exhaustion Phase (Figure 9A)

"Completely exhausted afternoon sleeper"

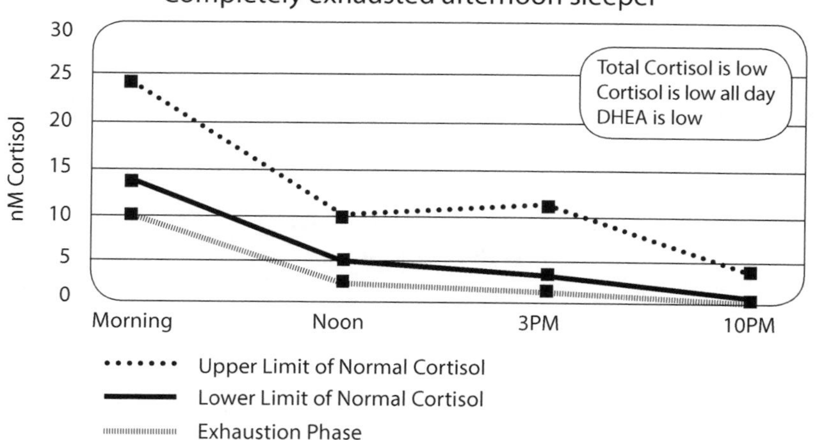

During this phase, which occurs after the adrenals have gone through the previous phases of alarm and resistance, is where the adrenals are unable to manufacture the cortisol and other hormones needed for daily function. We call this "adrenal burnout." It is still reversible, but more work is needed here to repair the adrenals.

Due to the severity of the headaches and chronicity of the condition, I found that certain medications and injections were often beneficial for symptom relief and the prevention of further attacks (see Chapter 14). However, it was important to combine the approaches — manage the pain by wisely utilizing prescription medications, while simultaneously working with the patient to balance the mind and body using a systems-based approach.

Determining the State of the Adrenals

I recommend and use a four-point cortisol saliva test to check my patients' cortisol output. I have found it to be the best measure currently available to adequately assess the presence of adrenal fatigue. In the absence of stress, the adrenals maintain a daily cortisol rhythm that peaks in the morning, lowers at midday, drops again in the afternoon, and falls to its lowest point before bed, allowing sleep to occur. Checking cortisol levels at each of these intervals throughout the day provides the most accurate snapshot of current stress hormone production levels. The results, which are denoted by stages, explain it all:

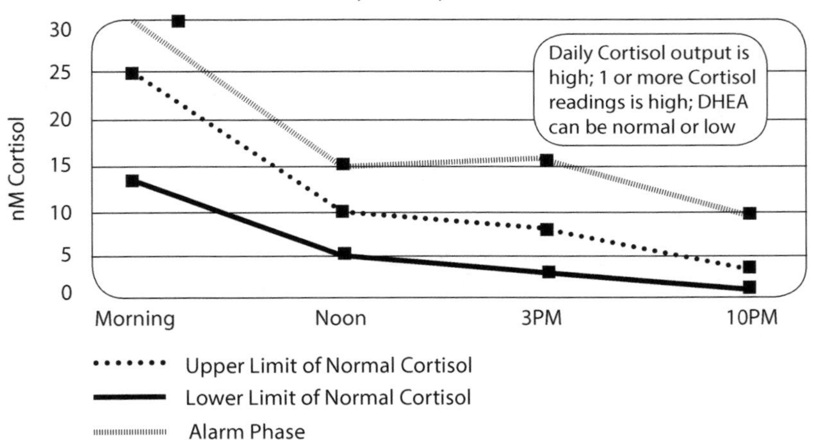

During this stage, the adrenals, due to input from the hypothalamus signaling chronic stress, release high levels of cortisol, along with the other adrenal hormones to help the mind and body handle the stress.

Common Cortisol Ranges — Resistance Phase (Figure 8A)

"Fatigued in the morning, difficulty sleeping at night"

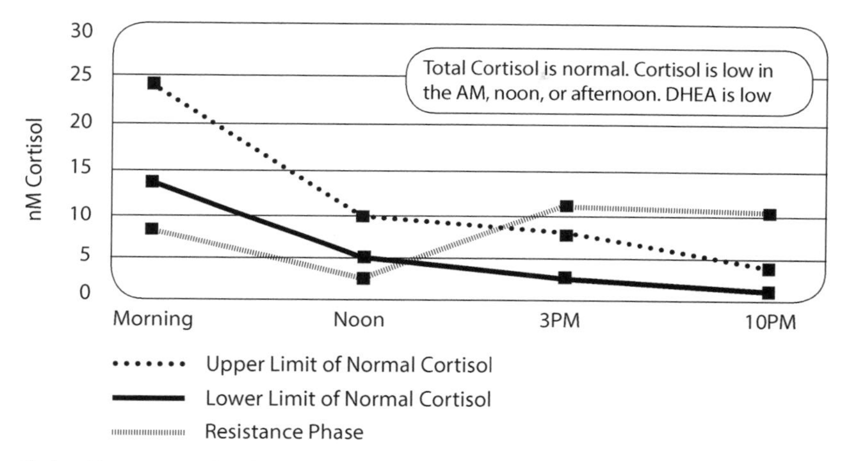

During this stage, since the adrenals have been "on" for too long, the adrenals start to fatigue, thus releasing less epinephrine and cortisol. Since it seems that the adrenals will not turn off soon, the hypothalamus starts to become desensitized to the ongoing stress response.

Common Cortisol Ranges — Exhaustion Phase (Figure 9A)

"Completely exhausted afternoon sleeper"

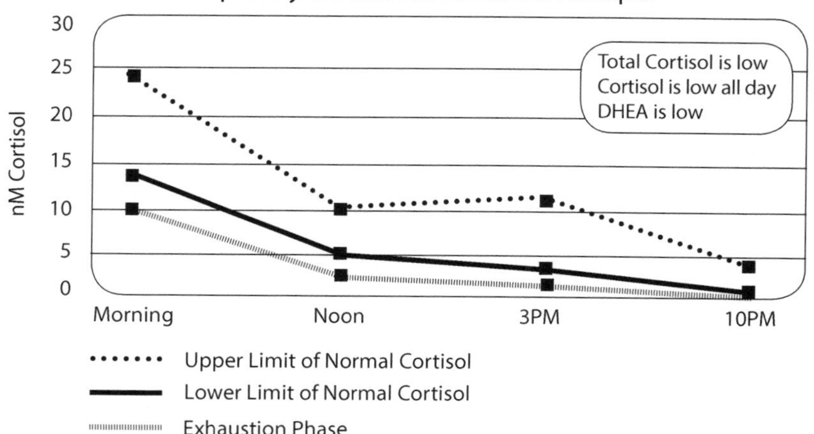

During this phase, which occurs after the adrenals have gone through the previous phases of alarm and resistance, is where the adrenals are unable to manufacture the cortisol and other hormones needed for daily function. We call this "adrenal burnout." It is still reversible, but more work is needed here to repair the adrenals.

Based on the adrenal test results of 83 patients in my clinic, I found 4% of patients in stage 1, 47% of patients in stage 2, 35% of patients in stage 3, and 5% of patients in stage 4. These findings demonstrate that slightly more than 90% of the patients suffering from migraine headaches were also in one of the four stages of adrenal fatigue, most in stage 2 or 3, which is moderate adrenal exhaustion. Why is this and what can be done to fix it?

For many patients, their in utero experience may have been stressed because their mothers may have suffered from various conditions, had a difficulty pregnancy, or had a complicated childbirth. Is it possible that one is born with a weaker, more vulnerable adrenal system that then became weaker due to stress, poor food choices, and an imbalanced lifestyle? Or maybe the adrenals were strong at birth, but a high level and intensity of stress exhausted the adrenal glands over time, leading to the current state?

The Adrenal-Thyroid Link

One of the most challenging clinical conundrums is to figure out if someone is suffering with symptoms linked to weak adrenals or a weak thyroid system, or both. In both of these scenarios, symptoms can include, but are not limited to: fatigue, headaches, low moods, difficulty sleeping and pain. Specific features such as a low body temperature, low pulse rate, or hair loss, especially of the outer portion of the eyebrow, can be clues to a thyroid dysfunction. The fascinating piece is that our body, since it operates as a system, is always trying to keep the adrenal rhythm and thyroid hormone production in balance.

An important concept we need to keep in mind, as depicted in the picture (Figure 10), is that our adrenal system and thyroid output are always working in unison. The best analogy to this I have heard comes from a very wise Dr. Janet Lang, during a 2007 lecture. She said to imagine yourself sitting at a stop light. Your foot is on the brake and your car is on, but you are at rest. Compare this state to the normal operation of your thyroid glands. They provide the "basal metabolic rate" in my view. They allow the body to take care of daily housekeeping tasks of maintaining cellular function, body temperature and appropriate energy utilization. Then the light turns green. What happens? At that point, your foot hits the accelerator and your car moves. This is how your adrenals function. When your mind tells them to "go" under stress, your car propels forward. At this time, your body starts to manufacture cortisol, rather than making thyroid hormone, since you need a hormone that will move you with more intensity. To keep our bodies in balance, we will not produce thyroid hormone when our cortisol levels increase. We choose to either be in a "basal metabolic mode" or a "go" mode. Your car cannot be at rest at a red light and accelerating during a green light at the same time, correct? How can we expect our thyroid and adrenals to work equally at the same time also? The system just does not operate that way. While one system is on, the other is taking rest.

Thus, if you find your thyroid production low, or you find your Free T4 or Free T3 to be reduced, you may want to consider how much stress your mind and body are under. The solution may lie in managing the stress, rather than trying to manage your thyroid.

Taking the Next Step

The common denominator for all imbalance is chronic stress. Applying the Ayurvedic model of doshas can help you understand the concept of living outside of your natural doshic state and how it can lead to imbalanced adrenal glands and hormone production. By following the recommended diet and lifestyle guidelines for your dosha type, you can restore the function of your adrenals, harmonize your body's circadian rhythms, and balance your system. Are you ready to enjoy life with less distress and less pain? Then let's gather another very important clue! Just turn the page to Chapter 7 to identify your Ayurvedic dosha and you'll be on the path to healing your discomfort and reclaiming your life.

The Interplay Between Adrenals, Thyroid and Stress (Figure 10)

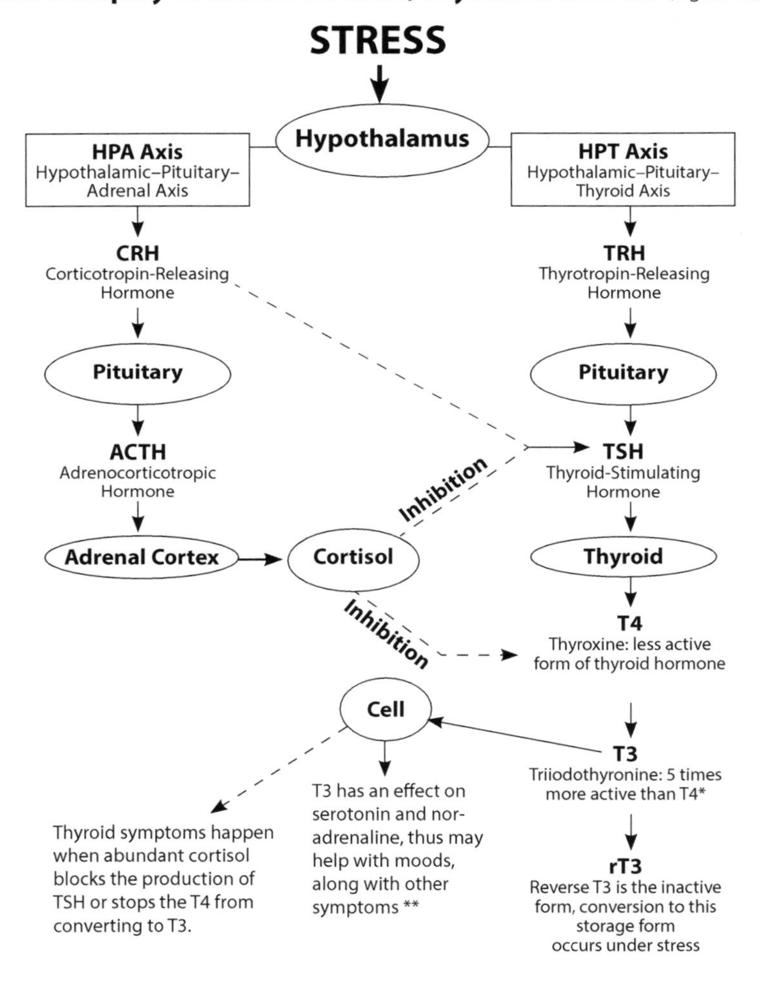

**HRT: The Answers. A Concise Guide for Solving the Hormone Replacement Therapy Puzzle.* Pamela Wartian Smith, MD, MPH

***The Thyroid Solution, A Revolutionary Mind-Body Program for Regaining Your Emotional and Physical Health*, Ridha Arem, MD

CHAPTER 7
The Dosha Test

"The only person you are destined to become is the person you decide to be."
Ralph Waldo Emerson

In conventional medicine, whatever is common for the majority of people is considered "normal." However, according to Dr. Vasant Lad, author of *Ayurveda — The Science of Self-healing*, in Ayurveda "normality must be evaluated individually, because every human constitution manifests its own particular and spontaneous temperament and functioning."[43]

Studying Ayurveda completely changed the way I looked at myself, family, patients, and friends. I was able to understand the tendencies that define our nature. Some are creative types and enthusiastic, some are more determined and focused, and others are more compassionate and relaxed. I was able to release thoughts and perceptions of people; instead of seeing them as inherently hyper, anxious, angry, or lazy, I began to view them as having a tendency toward an imbalanced dosha, which allowed me to view them in a more compassionate way. I was even able to better understand my own tendencies and emotional responses while under stress. For example, a relative whom I may have viewed as overly anxious and obsessive was perceived to be an individual with Vata excess. The patient who was easily angered by the front desk receptionist but also had a stern determination to "find an answer" to his pain is now easily understood as an individual with excessive Pitta in his physiology. The lethargic, depressed friend who couldn't lose weight falls into the Kapha imbalanced state.

Everyone has a specific dosha composition that is as unique as a fingerprint. Dr. Lad notes that this composition is comprised of all three types, with a predominant tendency toward one or more. The philosophy and science of Ayurveda provided me with greater insights on how to help my patients, as well as myself, to heal and understand the nature that drives us to be who we are.

The first requirement for you to become a partner in your healing is to understand your own dominant dosha, using the questionnaire that you'll find in this chapter. The beauty of Ayurveda is its simplicity. Once you're aware of your dosha, the key to health, happiness, and well-being is to adopt a lifestyle that maintains harmony and balance. I will admit that sometimes it is easier said than done, because many of us have become so imbalanced that the natural state of balance has been forgotten. Do not be distressed; we will unravel that mystery and find your ideal self. Ultimately, the goal is to help you make the best possible healthy choices for your daily life based on your body's needs.

Finding Your Dosha Type

Please answer the following questions to determine your dosha type. Circle the answer that best applies to you:

1. **My body weight/tendency is:**

    A. Thin, flexible, and/or loses weight easily
    B. Medium, muscular, and/or weight remains the same
    C. Heavy, gains weight easily

2. **My body frame is best described as:**

    A. Small-boned and/or flexible
    B. Medium bone structure and/or muscular
    C. Large build and solid

3. **My hair is generally:**

    A. Dry, brittle, and brown or black
    B. Oily, straight, premature graying/balding, blond or red hair
    C. Oily, thick and/or dark, healthy, and wavy

4. **My nose has the following features:**

    A. Uneven shape, deviated septum
    B. Long, pointed, may be red at tip
    C. Short and rounded

5. **My appetite is best described as:**
   A. Variable hunger — sometimes ravenous, sometimes not hungry. Tend to skip meals.
   B. Strong, sharp appetite. Can eat anything and need to eat often.
   C. Dull, steady appetite. Skipping meals doesn't have an effect.

6. **My joints are:**
   A. Prominent, bony protuberances, cracking, and/or popping
   B. Medium in size
   C. Rounded, well-covered (muscles/tissue cover joints), well-lubricated

7. **My body's temperature tolerance is such that I tend to feel:**
   A. Cold, with cold hands/feet and/or don't tolerate cold weather, prefer warm drinks
   B. Hot, may even feel flushed, prefer cool drinks, doesn't tolerate hot weather
   C. Worse in cool/damp weather

8. **My nails tend to be:**
   A. Dry, brittle
   B. Flexible and/or pink
   C. Thick and/or smooth

9. **My face is:**
   A. Oval
   B. Triangular (prominent jaw)
   C. Round

10. **My digestive tendency is:**
    A. Gas, constipation, and/or bloating
    B. Reflux, burning, and/or diarrhea
    C. Sluggish and/or forms mucus

11. In terms of my energy level:

A. I am always on the go; I start tasks and may have a hard time finishing them
B. I tend to think before I do; if I start a task, due to my organization/ intensity I will always finish
C. I am steady and calm; I do not like to rush, but when I start a task it will eventually get done

12. In terms of walking:

A. I walk fast
B. I am focused and determined when walking, but it's not necessarily fast
C. I walk calmly and slowly

13. My speech tends to be:

A. Very fast and sometimes unclear
B. Direct, clear, and precise
C. Slow, calm, and can be monotonous

14. My mind tends to be:

A. Creative, imaginative, restless, and/or emotional (moods may fluctuate)
B. Focused, sharp, efficient, and/or perfectionistic
C. Calm, relaxed, analytical, and/or slow

15. I often notice:

A. My energy level fluctuates in bursts
B. I am critical of myself and others, and/or stubborn
C. I am affectionate and forgiving

16. I would be best described as:

A. Lively, enthusiastic, and/or active; sometimes anxious
B. Organized, determined, and/or impatient; sometimes irritable
C. Calm, introspective, and/or lazy; sometimes depressed

17. If stress or conflict occurs, my mood or mind:

A. Changes quickly; I am prone to anxiety and find myself getting excitable
B. Changes slowly; I am prone to irritability and feel critical
C. Is mostly steady; it takes a lot to "ruffle my feathers," but I can become lazy and depressed

18. My decision making is:

A. Difficult since my mind vacillates
B. Quick, sometimes hasty
C. Slow with time taken to decide

19. My attention span is:

A. Short attention span and I do not have good focus
B. Long attention span with good focus, and I am detail oriented
C. Long attention span with good focus, and I am a "big picture" person

20. With sleep, I have:

A. Difficulty falling asleep and/or light and interrupted sleep
B. No problem falling asleep and sleep an average length; I may wake up in the middle of the night
C. No problem sleeping, sleep soundly, and usually have difficulty awakening

21. In regard to friendships:

A. I enjoy making and changing friends often
B. I keep a certain set of friends which may change due to jobs, locations, or schools
C. I have long-lasting, stable, and sincere friendships

22. With physical work or exercise, I tend to have:

A. Low tolerance with easy fatigue
B. Medium tolerance
C. High tolerance and very good endurance

Now, tally your answers and record the total number:

A. ________
B. ________
C. ________

If you have more "A" answers, your primary dosha type is Vata, and you'll find information about this dosha in Chapter 8. If you have more "B" answers, your primary dosha type is Pitta, and you can learn all about Pitta in Chapter 9. If you have more "C" answers, your dosha is Kapha. You'll find details in Chapter 10. What if your result totals are "2, 2, and 1"? See my blog: How to Understand Your Dosha — Interpreting the Quiz Results at www.ZiraMindAndBody.com/Interpret.

Thoroughly study your dominant dosha in the following chapters, and with these clues in hand you'll have a framework for closing the case on your headache pain and health challenges. You'll also enjoy learning more about the dosha types in your environment: spouse or significant other, children, parents, siblings, friends, and even co-workers. Welcome to a new way of understanding your health and your life!

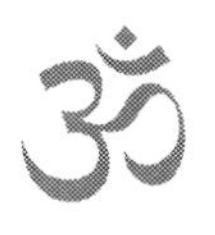

CHAPTER 8
Vata Dosha: Move Like the Wind

The Vata dosha provides the energy that controls bodily functions associated with motion, including blood circulation, breathing, blinking, and your heartbeat. When Vata dosha is balanced, you experience vitality and creativity. When Vata dosha is imbalanced, you have a tendency to experience anxiety and fear.[44]

Dr. Vasant Lad

I will never forget the conversation I had with my older sister Dipti a few years back while moving my practice. My new office space had all of the bells and whistles — including a beautiful yoga studio, fancy carpeting, and gleaming hardwood floors. The design and construction took an immense amount of effort, planning, and budgeting. During the build-out, I continued to stay busy seeing patients, giving lectures, attending conferences, and developing new, integrative healing protocols.

One day, Dipti asked me a question: "What would happen if you just sat still and didn't do anything? Is that something you could do? How would standing still make you feel?"

Dipti is the kind of sister who rarely criticizes. In addition to her good intentions, she has a way of speaking that would never offend anyone. But when she shares her insights, Dipti's statements command attention. I thought deeply about what Dipti asked. Of course, I thought about it while still multitasking — in the midst of taking calls and reviewing patients' charts.

You guessed it — I am an unapologetic Vata. Let me make this clear, I was not born into a predominant Vata type. I have lived a Vata-provoking life, thus I have increased my Vata nature over the years. The Vata dosha is comprised of the elements of air and space, and is governed by movement. Because we are on the move, on the go, and attempt to do far too much (under the auspices of multitasking), this dosha-type becomes easily and chronically imbalanced. I believe the poor state of our nation's health is due to our collective, vitiated (imbalanced) Vata state.

The Vata Dosha Type Patient

It was a beautiful spring day in Chicago and I was starting my day in clinic when I met Julie for the first time. Julie, a vibrant-appearing woman in her mid-40s, came in wearing her running gear. With a physique that looked like a marathoner, she had a small frame and dark hair pulled back into a ponytail. She was very talkative and friendly as she was checked in and brought into my office. During her vitals and weight check, Julie complained to my medical assistant that she had been gaining weight recently around her belly and couldn't understand why since she was an avid runner.

After a few minutes of small talk, I began with my favorite starting thought: "Julie, tell me when you last felt truly healthy and optimal in your mind, body, and soul." Julie responded, "Well, that's a tough question, but I guess I started getting headaches in college." It is always fascinating to me how many of my patients start with the complaint that they think I want to hear as a neurologist. Since my specialty is headache, when I start with a question about optimal health the history usually starts with when the headaches began. Since I have realized over the years that headaches generally begin with dysfunction outside of the brain — before the brain starts to manifest pain — I generally probe more on this.

I noticed that Julie's health intake form listed constipation and bloating as an ongoing problem. With her small frame and thin body, Julie held her abdomen as she described her digestive issues. When I asked her when these problems began, her response was, "Oh, I have been constipated since I was a baby!" In terms of fatigue, another symptom with which she suffered, she informed me, "I do not know what it is like to not wake up feeling fatigued; maybe it is because I never sleep well!"

Julie had an exuberance to her that was quite engaging. She smiled and used her hands wildly to describe her trials and tribulations over the years. She was animated and very lively during this early part of the interview. After going back to my original question about when she last felt optimal, it was very clear to me that Julie had truly never felt optimal. With her early history of digestive issues and anxiety with school leading to insomnia and daily fatigue, the headaches came as a result of years of living out of balance.

Julie then began talking at a pace where I could barely keep up with my typing. Her speech was rapid and she jumped from one topic to another. She told me about the many doctors she saw when she was suffering with fatigue and began having headaches. These doctors prescribed medications which often made her feel "like a zombie" and gave her side effects. She made it very clear to me that she was sensitive to medications and I needed to be careful with her when prescribing them.

She began describing her headaches. Her pain started in her neck and then eventually moved to the back of her head. She was perplexed as to why the left side of her head and body seemed to be more often involved with pain than the right side. I noted that these clues are all indicative of the Vata dosha type.

She told me the conclusion most doctors made was, "You are just stressed and need to relax." Having two children and running a busy real estate company, she found the only way she knew how to relax was through exercise. In fact, most of the doctors she had seen had encouraged her to exercise in the manner she had been. Her routine included either a three-mile run or a cardio "boot camp" class daily. When I asked her how she would feel if she stopped exercising or just skipped a day, her response was, "I would feel horrible! I need to exercise, otherwise I wouldn't be able to survive." I asked her when her need to exercise daily began. She told me she had been exercising this way since she was in her teens, and her daily need to exercise began in her 20s. This was another clue, indicating when her adrenals went into fatigue. (See Chapter 6 for a detailed discussion of adrenal fatigue.)

She was sitting on the edge of her seat as she looked at me with bewilderment. She wanted to know why she had suffered and needed someone to figure out the mysterious onset of her headaches, which were now daily. To me, there was no mystery here. Her body had become imbalanced in one of the key doshic (mind-body) states and her attempt to keep her dosha in balance actually made her feel worse.

Julie, like many of my patients, is a classic Vata dosha type. Her mind-body type gives her the enthusiasm to keep moving and going. Because most of us do not know what the Vata diet involves, we often eat or drink in a way that provokes this state and causes digestive issues. (See Chapter 11 for a detailed discussion of diet.) When Vata individuals feel stressed, they love to move. They choose running, bicycling, and Vinyasa flow-type yoga classes. Meals are not eaten at regular times and the sleep routine is not well established. They often will fatigue their adrenals through their need to move and go, along with a lack of regularity in their routine. Living this way for years eventually creates symptoms that can then lead to the onset of many diseases.

Understanding the Vata Dosha Type

The Vata dosha type is comprised of air and space elements and is governed by movement. Because you are always on the go and attempt to do far too much (under the auspices of multitasking), your dosha type becomes easily and chronically imbalanced. I believe the poor state of our nation's health is due to our collective, vitiated (imbalanced) Vata state.

To keep up with the frenetic pace that Vata dosha types create, you most often skip breakfast. You are classic multitaskers, rushing to work or activities while talking on the phone, quickly eating lunch (if at all), and hurrying throughout the day. With the advent of high-speed internet, 24/7 online access, texting, emailing, tweeting, and the growing addiction to the cell phone, Vatas rarely make the time to shut off the outside world. God forbid you forget to charge your cell phone or *consciously* turn it off for an hour! Could you be away from your phone that long? If a text comes in or your cell phone rings, buzzes, or vibrates, do you find yourself quickly responding to every call or text?

The ever-present and growing health challenge for the Vata dosha type is that your ability to disconnect is being arrested. As such, your system is chronically in a state of movement (and needing constant activation and stimulation). What happens to your brain and body in this chronic state? It can lead to adrenal fatigue, a time when your adrenal glands are unable to keep up with the body's demands for the necessary hormones norepinephrine, epinephrine, cortisol, and DHEA without the adequate precursors and vitamins. The mind also suffers in this state of Vata imbalance. Depleted adrenals can lead to racing thoughts, anxiety, panic, insomnia (especially difficulty falling asleep), and difficulty focusing.

I have had many patients who were previously diagnosed with difficulty in focusing when their problems actually stemmed from an imbalanced Vata dosha type. These patients responded positively to stimulant medications, such as dextroamphetamine sulfate (also known as Adderall) and Vyvanse, which, interestingly, increase norepinephrine and dopamine levels. Remember that when adrenals are turned on for too long they become fatigued. During this time, the production of norepinephrine and epinephrine decreases. We do, at times, need to use medications. I find that it is also important to remember that dietary and lifestyle changes can be utilized to balance this state. By using a comprehensive approach, we may be better equipped to manage and possibly resolve the symptoms at hand.

While all dosha types need to be concerned about hydration, this is a critical issue for Vata dosha types. It's essential that you stay well-hydrated with water. Dehydration further imbalances the Vata (dry) state. Signs of dehydration include dry mouth, fatigue, dark-colored urine, dry skin, headache, constipation, and dizziness or lightheadedness.

Vata Dosha Type Headaches

To understand the Vata dosha type headache, think of wind blowing through your body — it makes you feel cold and dry and can lead to mind spinning. The following are characteristics of the Vata dosha type headache:

- Location of the pain is usually the occipital or base of the skull
- Pain can have a quality of a tight band around head or throbbing in nature
- Sensitivity to medications
- Associated features include seizures and/or auras
- Mood symptoms include restlessness, difficulty focusing, and anxiety
- Digestive issues include gas, bloating, and constipation
- Triggers for pain include eating Vata-provoking foods (cold, dry), skipping meals, lack of sleep, travel, overexertion, suppressing emotion, and overexercising.[45]

Take the following quiz to see if the symptoms you are experiencing are the result of Vata dosha type imbalance. Check all of the symptoms that best describe your experience:

___ Left-sided pain
___ Discomfort of the neck or back of head
___ Dizziness
___ Mind racing or restless thoughts
___ Gas, bloating, or constipation
___ Feeling dry and cold
___ Very sensitive to weather shifts or travel
___ Lack of regular schedule (sleep and meal times vary daily)
___ Talking excessively or very fast (ask your family!)
___ Problems falling asleep
___ Sensitive to sound
___ **Total number of items checked**

If you checked more than two items, your Vata dosha type is in an imbalanced state. The more items checked, the more imbalanced the state.

Dietary and Lifestyle Choices for Balancing the Vata Dosha

The key to healing an imbalanced Vata dosha is to make dietary and lifestyle changes. Medication may also be required to control the severity of symptoms.

Sweet fruits, small beans, rice, all nuts (preferably soaked first or toasted/roasted), and dairy products are good choices for Vata dosha types. Please note that you may have an asymptomatic intolerance to dairy products, which can only be determined with testing. Until you know for sure, consider using almond or rice milk as a substitute. For some people, boiling milk is also non-reactive. Vata dosha types should:

- Start with warm, cooked, and easily-digestible foods
- Sauté or steam vegetables
- Make blended or whole-vegetable soups
- Avoid raw and crunchy foods

For more information on choosing foods to balance the Vata dosha, see Chapter 11.

Lifestyle habits are also an integral component in balancing the Vata dosha. Following are some recommendations that you can implement in your daily routine to help restore your vitality. Which of these can you start incorporating in your life today?

- Establish a consistent routine. Wake up and go to bed at the same time each day. An ideal bedtime is 10 p.m.
- Eat three regularly-scheduled meals daily, with lunch being the largest and most important meal.
- Meditate or practice yoga three times per week.
- *Slow down!* Take time to finish each task prior to moving on to the next. Keep multitasking to a minimum.
- Stay hydrated. Consume one-half of your body weight in water every day. For example, a person weighing 140 pounds should drink a minimum of 70 ounces of water. Monitor yourself for signs of dehydration.
- Begin a daily practice of *Abhyanga*, a therapeutic self-massage using unrefined sesame seed oil on the head and body. The benefits of Abhyanga, also referred to as "self-abhy," include increased circulation, calming of the nerves, increased mental alertness, and deeper sleep.
- Eat a Vata dosha type balancing diet, adding appropriate seasonings and spices.
- Whenever possible, dine in a calm, relaxed atmosphere. Chew slowly and completely when eating. Do your best to take at least 30 minutes for lunch.
- Limit or remove caffeine from the diet.

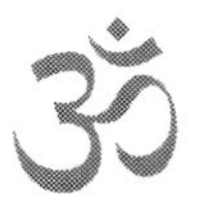

CHAPTER 9
Pitta Dosha: Rage Like Fire

The Pitta dosha provides the energy that controls the body's metabolic systems, including digestion and absorption of nutrients, along with serving as the source of your body's temperature. When the Pitta dosha is in balance, you experience contentment and intelligence. When Pitta is out of balance, you have a hard time controlling anger and can be prone to ulcers.[46]

Dr. Vasant Lad

I still remember walking to the front of the auditorium to accept the "hardest worker" award. I was in sixth grade and I was mortified. I felt a surge of embarrassment as I walked back to my seat. Why did I feel that way? Wasn't it better to be a "hard worker" than "most popular" or "best dressed"?

It's still fascinating to me how this memory remains vivid and palpable after all of these years. I think it's because working hard seems to be part of my genetics, or should I say "energetics." From getting my education to opening my own business, setting goals and working hard to accomplish those goals is how I've always lived my life.

The Pitta Dosha Type Patient

Living in Chicago, I have become comfortable with the fact that the weather will often be unpredictable. It was a hot day in late September when many of us thought fall had arrived, but to our surprise it suddenly felt like the middle of the summer.

Martin was an attractive man in his mid-50s. As he walked into the office, he told my staff that he had a business meeting in an hour and wanted to make sure I was running on schedule. He maintained a stern look and criticized my medical assistant when she asked him for his paperwork. He insisted that he did not receive our customary email reminding him to fill out paperwork before his initial appointment, and with haste he grabbed the blank intake forms. He sat in the waiting room and quickly began filling out the forms. My team alerted me about his time restraints and the fact that paperwork (which is lengthy) was not completed before the visit. I had a feeling that I knew where this visit was going to take us.

As I brought Martin back to my office, I offered him a glass of water. He responded that he was fine as he already had his coffee on his way to the clinic. "Oh, I am in trouble," I thought. I know what caffeine does to the Pitta types. I gently asked, "What brings you in today?" Martin replied with no hesitation, "My head has been out of control over the last few months and we need to do something about it!" I always love how physicians are brought into the sufferers' world. Don't get me wrong, I have plenty of compassion for my patients. I find it interesting how much emphasis we place on the physician to do the work rather than realizing that it is the patient, not the physician, who needs to put forth the effort in order for the system to heal. I learned that Martin was having near-daily migraines around 3 p.m. in the afternoon and was unable to work productively over the last few months.

I then began asking him about his digestion and lifestyle. "Martin, when do you have lunch and how is your digestion?" Martin took a moment to ponder this. "Well, I seem to have a lot of burning after I eat, but an antacid usually takes care of that, so I wouldn't consider that a problem. I tend to run to the bathroom more frequently than I would like to admit when I eat poorly or am under stress." I then asked him about his digestive system in relation to attacks of pain. Martin replied, "I always get nauseated when I have a migraine. I take nausea medications but they make me tired. At times, I vomit and then it is interesting as my headache is usually better after this." For those with a Pitta tendency, we find symptoms such as heartburn, nausea, and diarrhea to be common complaints. These symptoms signify excess "heat" in the digestive system. In fact, it is believed that vomiting, especially with migraine attacks, is the body's natural way of removing this excess "heat." Thus, I wasn't surprised that Martin's head pain improved after vomiting.

I learned that Martin often skips lunch or conducts intense business meetings during the lunch hour. In regard to Ayurvedic digestion, the most important meal of the day is lunch. When the sun is at its peak, we release the greatest amount of digestive enzymes and our body is prepared to break down foods to nourish our system. If we skip meals or, almost worse, have stressful, intense meetings during this time, we are very likely to have excess heat symptoms later in the day. This style of eating (or not eating!) explained why Martin was prone to afternoon migraines. In addition, he often chose hot and spicy foods, which are known to be heat inducing and are not recommended for Pitta types.

Finally, we discussed exercise. One of Martin's favorite forms of exercise was intense cardio at the gym with his trainer. We had a long conversation about trying to create balance in life. If he lives life with intensity during the day while working, he needs to spend his off hours doing something quieting and mindful, such as meditation and yoga. Martin decided he would start a restorative yoga practice.

Martin is a classic Pitta type who has found himself in an imbalanced state with this dosha. His mind is critical and demanding, with a touch of arrogance. With this energy of the mind, he conducts intense business meetings, often skipping lunch, which is the most important meal for his type. His "off time" is spent exercising intensely, which only increases his fire-state imbalance. By carefully choosing Pitta-balancing foods and herbals and by making lifestyle changes, Martin saw that his headaches and digestive symptoms improved over time. He also found his mind becoming more compassionate and pleasant, which was nice for not only himself but everyone around him.

Understanding the Pitta Dosha Type

According to Ayurveda, the elements of fire and water come together to create the Pitta dosha type, which — if you haven't guessed it by now — is my primary dosha type. Pitta governs metabolism and generates heat in the body. It is this dosha type that fuels your ability to accomplish your goals, make decisions, and take action. Without the fire state, tasks are difficult to complete.

For Pitta dosha type individuals, speaking and lecturing are a passion. They love to speak their minds with passion, give instruction, and teach strategic concepts. Outlining a plan and completing a task list is something Pittas love to do, and they are naturals at it. So, how can this driven state lead to an imbalance?

Working hard is the cornerstone of the Westernized model of success. To succeed in life requires productivity, right? For those whose families risked their lives to bring us to the United States, hard work is the drumbeat to which we march through life. But at some point, that driven, heated, charged lifestyle begins to lose momentum. It is virtually impossible to stay in the Pitta state for too long before becoming symptomatic.

The symptoms of excessive Pitta include anger, irritability, migraines, feeling hot, difficulty staying asleep, and digestive issues such as reflux and diarrhea. The hard-driving, perfectionistic Pitta dosha type can push the adrenals to exhaustion and deplete hormones, just like an imbalanced Vata state. I have often found adrenal fatigue to be a core challenge for those with Pitta dosha types. As a matter of fact, a research study focusing on chronic headache patients found that adolescents with chronic headaches were more likely to be perfectionistic.[47] The low hormone state (of depleted adrenal glands) can exacerbate feelings of anger and contribute to mood swings. If left unbalanced, it can lead to potential nutrient and neurotransmitter depletion.

Pitta Dosha Type Headaches

To understand the Pitta dosha type headache, think of increasing fire, leading to heat and increased metabolic activity. The following are characteristics of the Pitta dosha type headache:

- The location of the pain is usually the temples and behind the eyes. Pain presents itself as burning, sharp, and intense, especially if the pain is on the right side of the head.
- Moderate to severe in nature
- Medication issues can lead to nausea, reflux (burning sensation), and/or diarrhea
- Associated features include nausea, vomiting, and light sensitivity
- Mood symptoms include uncontrolled anger and mood swings
- Digestive issues include reflux and diarrhea[48]

Isn't it interesting that Ayurveda links these headaches to a state of increased inflammation? Triggers for pain include exposure to heat, spicy foods, excessive demands, extremely high-pressure situations, and skipping lunch. Ayurveda may offer clarity about which patients may be the best candidates for modern-day treatment modalities.

Take the following quiz to see if the symptoms you are experiencing are the result of Pitta dosha type imbalance. Check all of the symptoms that best describe your experience:

___ Right-sided location of symptoms
___ Discomfort in temples, behind/above the eyes
___ Associated with burning
___ Short-fused or edgy moods
___ Problems staying asleep
___ Sensitivity to light
___ Intolerance to heat
___ Vertigo (spinning room)
___ Diarrhea or reflux
___ Nausea or vomiting
___ **Total number of items checked**

If you checked more than two items, your Pitta dosha type is in an imbalanced state. The more items checked, the more imbalanced the state.

Dietary and Lifestyle Choices for Balancing the Pitta Dosha

The key to healing an imbalanced Pitta dosha is to make dietary and lifestyle changes. Pitta dosha types should:

- Choose fresh vegetables and fruits that are watery and sweet, such as cherries, cucumbers, melons, and avocado.
- Have lots of salads with dark greens such as arugula, dandelion, and kale.
- Avoid fried and spicy foods.

For more information on choosing foods to balance the Pitta dosha, see Chapter 11.

Lifestyle habits are also an integral component in balancing the Pitta dosha. Following are some recommendations that you can implement in your daily routine to help restore your vitality. Which of these can you start incorporating in your life today?

- Eat all meals on a regular schedule, especially lunch. You should never skip lunch.

- Go to bed no later than 10 p.m. The Pitta window for detoxification of the liver occurs between 10 p.m. and 2 a.m. Sleeping during this time allows the mind and body to detoxify, cleanse, and reset.
- Laugh hard and laugh often! Pittas need to learn to relax and enjoy life. Don't take everything so seriously.
- Practice gentle exercises, such as restorative yoga and meditation. Avoid hot yoga or intense workouts.
- Follow a Pitta dosha type balancing diet.

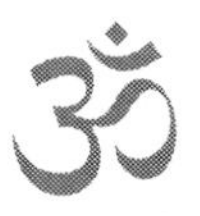

CHAPTER 10

Kapha Dosha: The Dosha of Groundedness

The Kapha dosha provides the energy that controls the body's growth. It supplies water to all of the body's parts, moisturizes the skin, and maintains the immune system. When the Kapha dosha is in balance, you're easy-going and relaxed. When Kapha is out of balance, you are prone to greed, depression and envy.

Dr. Vasant Lad

Think about the people with whom you feel relaxed the moment you see them. They are never in a rush and always speak calmly. More than likely, these individuals are Kapha dosha type. Given the frenetic pace of our lifestyle, finding people with this unique disposition is becoming more challenging because there seems to be so little time to slow down, reflect, and be still. For most of us, making time for calm and quiet is now considered a luxury; we only do it when we're on vacation or ill. However, the mind can only clearly process thoughts, feelings, and beliefs when it is uncluttered. Slowing down is now a necessity.

The Kapha Dosha Type Patient

Spring is a time of renewal and usually brings excitement after a long, cold winter. For certain patients, this is the time of year when their symptoms become intolerable. Liz was one of those individuals. Liz was one of the kindest patients in our practice. She was soft spoken, kind, and always seemingly calm even when she wasn't feeling optimal. While she was being checked in, my medical assistant noted a five-pound weight gain from her previous visit. Liz seemed a bit depressed and was not her usual self during the intake.

After we sat down and sipped on our tea, I asked Liz, "How are you doing today? You seem a bit distraught." Liz looked down at her hands and paused. Then she looked up and told me that she had been feeling unwell for a few months now. "I have been feeling so tired and sluggish. I wake up congested and think I may be depressed. I am not sure why I am feeling this way," she explained.

Our last visit was six months prior, and things had taken a turn over the last three months. She had wanted to come in sooner but didn't feel motivated to call, even though she knew that she needed treatment. To comfort herself, Liz began eating foods such as cookies, cakes, and cheese. These seemed to be mood lifting for her. She had seen her primary care physician, who recommended some allergy medications and sinus sprays to relieve her congestion. "The allergy medications make me tired and the sprays do help with my congestion, but I need them every day. Is this ok?" she asked.

I am always perplexed with questions such as these. Is it ok to require a medication to suppress symptoms that are occurring daily? According to Ayurvedic literature, the purpose of a symptom is to identify which system or dosha is imbalanced and to correct the imbalance, not cover it with a medication. Allergy medication or nasal sprays are not generally a problem if taken short term. My concern was with addressing the cause of the congestion, not just the symptoms. In addition, she admitted to not exercising in months.

Liz is a classic Kapha type who has gone into imbalance with the season shift, along with her lack of exercise and consumption of heavy foods. We recommended some cleansing herbals and teas, along with a vigorous yoga and pranayama (breath) exercise to be done daily in order to help her reduce her Kapha excess.

Understanding the Kapha Dosha Type

In college, as my Pitta nature drove me to study hard and stay focused on my goals, I was sometimes envious of my Kapha friends. Although their laid-back manner made it easy for me to write them off as lazy, there was a part of me that wished I knew how to be more relaxed. Looking back, they may have wished they could have been more driven. True Kapha dosha types, however, prefer to relax and think; they are uncomfortable being pushed to do too much.

Kapha, which is composed of earth and water elements, creates structure, groundedness, and stability. If this is your dominant dosha type, you have a natural ability to stay calm and relaxed, even under duress. Kapha dosha types tend to be more compassionate and generous than other doshas, and they can easily become attached.

In contrast to those with a Vata dosha type, who are always moving, Kaphas are generally sitting still. In balance, Kapha dosha types tend to think in a slow, analytical manner and make wise decisions. They have endurance and can handle stress with poise and finesse.

The challenge for Kapha dosha types is their tendency to gain weight, creating a "heavy" mind and body. The mind can become tired, apathetic, and depressed. In the extreme, they tend to be "couch potatoes." Wet, cold, and rainy or snowy days also can make everyone feel more Kapha-like.

Kapha Dosha Type Headaches

To understand the Kapha dosha type headache, think of feeling grounded and rooted to the earth with a mind that stays even and calm, unless it gets too heavy and depressed. The following are characteristics of the Kapha dosha type headache:

- Location of the pain is usually frontal
- Nature of headache is mild to moderate intensity
- Medication issues include fatigue or heaviness
- Associated features include congestion, allergies, and weight gain
- Mood symptoms include low moods, lack of energy, and feeling sluggish
- Digestive issues include feeling "heavy" after meals

Triggers for pain include inactivity, eating heavy foods (dairy), eating cold leftover foods, and damp weather.

Take the following quiz to see if the symptoms you are experiencing are the result of Kapha dosha type imbalance. Check all of the symptoms that best describe your experience:

___ Discomfort in a frontal location
___ Worse with bending down
___ Sinus congestion
___ Allergies
___ Depression
___ Feeling unmotivated
___ Gaining weight
___ Tendency to oversleep
___ Sensitive to smell
___ **Total number of items checked**

If you checked more than two items, your Kapha dosha type is in an imbalanced state. The more items checked, the more imbalanced the state.

Dietary and Lifestyle Choices for Balancing the Kapha Dosha

The key to healing an imbalanced Kapha dosha is to make dietary and lifestyle changes. Maintaining dietary balance is a challenge for Kapha dosha types. Kapha dosha types should:

- Choose foods that are light, warm, and spicy.
- Avoid heavy oil and processed sugars, both of which are detrimental.
- Avoid heavy foods, especially dairy products.
- Use lots of spices such as black pepper, ginger, cumin, chili, and lots of bitter, dark greens.

For more information on choosing foods to balance the Kapha dosha, see Chapter 11.

Lifestyle habits are also an integral component in balancing the Kapha dosha. Following are some recommendations that you can implement in your daily routine to help restore your vitality. Which of these can you start incorporating in your life today?

- Eat all meals on time.
- Kapha types tend to not feel hungry, so it is important to eat in order to regulate the circadian rhythm. Lunch should be the largest meal.
- Avoid foods that contribute to Kapha dosha type imbalance, such as oily, fried, and processed foods.

- Exercise daily. Vigorous exercise is important for building heat (and increasing metabolism). In yoga, choose poses that are Kapha dosha type balancing, such as "dancing Shiva."
- Arise daily at 6 a.m. The time between 6-10 a.m. is considered the Kapha time of the morning, and sleeping into this window of time can lead to excess sleepiness and fatigue (Kapha symptoms) into the day hours.
- Avoid napping, as it can disturb your circadian rhythm.
- Drink teas that warm the body and stimulate the mind — Kapha CCF tea or teas with clove and ginger.

PART III:
Close the Case

CHAPTER 11
Eat for Your Dosha Type

"At the center of your being you have the answer; you know who you are and you know what you want."
Lao Tzu

As a self-declared "foodie," I will readily admit that I love to eat. My mother, who worked as a home economics teacher in Uganda, had a passion for cooking. A Pitta dosha type, she incorporated spices and combined foods in ways that I could never imagine. She had an extraordinary ability to look inside the refrigerator and pull out random items, such as beets, cauliflower, cilantro, sprouted mung beans, and lemon juice, and turn it into the most delectable salad. After eating her rich, flavorful meals, often in small portions, I still recall feeling full and satisfied. When I compare those dining experiences to more recent years when I have had bountiful American meals which left me feeling dissatisfied, I would ask myself, "Why did my mom's cooking leave me feeling much more energetic and vibrant than the other meals I have eaten?"

It took me years to realize this simple truth: my mother, using her vast knowledge and wide array of foods, spices, and flavors, had the uncanny ability to honor the importance of satisfying the body's six tastes. Based on the principles of Ayurveda, every meal you eat should incorporate six tastes: sweet, salty, sour, bitter, pungent, and astringent. The American diet is notorious for its special attention to sweet, sour, and salty. Without incorporating the bitter, pungent, and astringent tastes, your stomach feels dissatisfied. Without the six tastes, you also don't have the capacity to digest food very well. At the end of this chapter you'll find a chart outlining each of the six tastes, the source of each taste, and the effect each has on your dosha. But first, it's important that you understand cravings and how they impact your health.

According to statistics released by the American Heart Association in 2013, more than half of the nation's adults over age 20 are overweight or obese. Obesity has now been linked as a modifiable risk factor to the development of chronic migraines.[49] Close to 24 million children between the ages of 2 and 19 are overweight or obese, which can only lead to a greater risk of obesity-related diagnoses such as diabetes.[50]

Michael Moss, an award-winning investigative reporter for the *New York Times*, is the author of an important book about our nation's burgeoning health crisis, *Salt Sugar Fat*. He reports:

> *So why are the diabetes and obesity and hypertension numbers still spiraling out of control? It's not just a matter of poor willpower on the part of the consumer and a give-the-people-what-they-want attitude on the part of the food manufacturers. What I found, over four years of research and reporting, was a conscious effort — taking place in labs and marketing meetings and grocery-store aisles — to get people hooked on foods that are convenient and inexpensive.*[51]

Cravings for salt, sugar, and fat often drive you to desire certain foods, and I believe the cravings that make you feel out of control (sweet or salty, in particular) stem from an imbalanced dosha type, as well as biochemical imbalances.

Eating the foods you crave briefly pacifies the mind. For example, a Vata dosha type may feed anxiety by eating sweet foods. Sweet balances the Vata dosha. The problem is that these foods stimulate an adrenal "flight or fight" reaction, leading to elevated cortisol, an increase in insulin, and an increase in fat deposits. The body builds its wall of protection (extra weight) around the waistline. The craving for carbohydrates increases in order to maintain adequate blood sugar levels. If you satiate those cravings with processed food, your blood sugar will spike and then drop quickly, launching the cycle all over again. At the same time, when you restrict foods or tastes that your body needs, you also activate a craving cycle.

Although no clinical studies have been reported linking low blood sugar to migraine headaches, many migraine patients explain that they feel dizzy or light-headed prior to or during an attack. Supporting the adrenal glands or adding more lean protein to the diet can help pacify these symptoms.

Another known trigger to the development of a migraine is skipping meals. Any patient who has migraines, particularly those who are Pitta dosha type, should never skip a meal, especially lunch. During the hours of 10 a.m. and 2 p.m. is when the body releases the most digestive enzymes and hydrochloric acid needed to break down foods and extract nutrients your body can use. Skipping lunch deprives the body and the brain of much-needed nourishment.

By making mindful eating your way of life, you can help facilitate your body's ability to overcome headaches, insomnia, moods issues, and more. Here are some essential steps to keep in mind:

- Make lunch your largest meal of the day.
- Limit the amount of fluid you drink while eating.
- Do your best to chew slowly, and stay calm while eating.
- Plan to complete dinner before 7:30 p.m.

The goal of incorporating dietary information in your program to improve your symptoms is to help you *expand* your focus to improve your overall health. In Ayurveda, foods are used medicinally to treat physical imbalances, and herbs are used to help the mind and body work in concert on a deeper, more subtle level.[52] Foods can be either medicinal or toxic, meaning they support or disrupt the body's digestive system. A disrupted and imbalanced system is more prone to produce many neurological symptoms.

Because each of us has a unique mind-body type, it's important to make sure that the foods eaten are based on our specific mind-body type *and* the season. During the cold and dry winter months, it's important to eat warm and grounding foods that are well-oleated (prepared with ghee or healthy fats). During the intense heat of summer, our bodies need cooling foods such as watermelon, cilantro, and coconut juice.

Be sure that your diet incorporates the following six tastes, based on your dosha type, which will satisfy each of the body's nutritional needs for fats, proteins, carbohydrates, water, vitamins, and minerals.

Taste	Source	Impact on Doshas
Sweet	Fruit, grains, pasta, wheat, starchy vegetables, dairy, sugar, agave, honey, molasses	Balances Vata and Pitta doshas Aggravates Kapha dosha
Sour	Citrus fruits, berries, tomatoes, vinegar, fermented foods, salad dressing, alcohol	Balances Vata dosha Aggravates Pitta and Kapha doshas
Salty	Sea salt, wheat-free soy sauce, sea vegetables, salted meats or fish	Balances Vata dosha Aggravates Kapha and Pitta doshas
Pungent	Peppers, chilies, onions, garlic, cayenne, black pepper, cloves, ginger, mustard, spicy spices, salsa	Balances Kapha dosha Aggravates Vata and Pitta doshas
Bitter	Dark green leafy vegetables, green and yellow vegetables, kale, celery, broccoli, sprouts, beets	Balances Pitta and Kapha doshas Aggravates Vata dosha
Astringent	Lentils, dried beans, raw fruits, cauliflower, pomegranates, tea, herbs	Balances Pitta and Kapha doshas Aggravates Vata dosha

The most important concept to remember is to choose foods based on your dosha type and the season. Listen to your body and respond appropriately to the signals. If you experience fatigue, bloating, pain, mood changes, or an impact on your ability to sleep after eating a particular food, your body is letting you know that it's out of balance.

Restoring your balance is crucial to reversing the trajectory of poor health and headaches. Along with choosing the right foods, detoxification is another action step you can take to facilitate balance. Let's take a look at detoxification in the next chapter and continue solving the mystery of your ailments!

CHAPTER 12

Detoxification of the Body and Mind

"Health is a state of complete harmony of the body, mind, and spirit. When one is free from physical disabilities and mental distractions, the gates of the soul open."

B.K.S. Iyengar

One of the unique aspects about the healing art of Ayurveda is its emphasis on the importance of detoxification. You may have previously heard about detoxification in the context of weight-loss programs. However, the purpose of detoxification in Ayurveda is to restore balance.

It is important to understand the concept of "toxin" as it is used in integrative medicine. Toxins are any substance that create imbalance in your health or well-being. A toxin in the body can be caused by poor dietary choices, food intolerances, stress, unfiltered water, alcohol, food additives, genetically-modified foods, or pollutants in the home or in the environment.

One of the most common toxins to which you may currently be exposed on a daily basis is called "paraben." Parabens are contained in personal care products, such as skin cleansers and shampoo, and are used to prevent the growth of fungus and bacteria. Have you noticed an increase in "paraben-free" labeling and wondered what that meant? Parabens are known to mimic hormones in the body, particularly estrogen. A 2004 study conducted by Dr. Phillipa Darbre, a researcher in biomolecular sciences at the University of Reading in England, found a link between parabens and breast cancer.[53] While the study did not conclude that parabens caused cancer, researchers were alarmed to find the preservative in the cancer cells of breast tumors.[54]

Certain toxins are now referred to as "obesogens" because they literally alter the body's metabolism, fat cell development, and hormonal function, and they impact appetite.[55] The list of "obesogens" includes many popular food ingredients, such as high fructose corn syrup and soy.[56] This issue is one of the most frightening we currently face in the United States. Obesity rates are higher than ever, especially for children. It's important that you understand the detoxification process not only for yourself, but for the health and well-being of your children.

Unless the toxins are regularly removed from the system, it can lead to a toxic buildup that can manifest as physical and/or emotional disorders or disease. Keep in mind that as you age, the body's natural mechanisms for removing toxins from the system are not as effective, which increases the need for regular detoxification.

How Do You Detoxify?

Before I explain the Ayurvedic mode of detoxification, let's discuss the systems involved in detoxification. Your body has an elaborate structure for digesting and using nourishment, as well as for expelling what is not needed. The lymphatic system transports toxins from the venous system to the exit organs, which include your liver, digestive tract, kidneys, and skin.

Most people don't realize that the skin is the primary "window" used to evaluate health because it is one of the body's largest exit organs. During a recent family trip to London and Paris, I had a first-hand experience of my skin representing what was going on inside my body. During our stay, I decided to eat like the Europeans instead of maintaining the gluten- and dairy-free regimen I maintain at home. I ate bread and cheese (how can you not have a croissant in Paris?). What was the result? Since I am a Pitta dosha type, I developed a small amount of acne on my right cheek and chin. These are the areas of the face associated with the digestive tract. I was very surprised, since I had not had an acne outbreak in years. Symptoms on the right side of the body are linked to Pitta dosha type imbalances if excess heat or inflammation is present, such as the acne on my face. Other manifestations of this state are rosacea, psoriasis, and hives. As soon as I returned home, I began my own detoxification process to restore my body's balance.

Sweat is another important method of detoxification, which causes the body to release toxins through the skin. In addition to exercise, another great way to sweat is using a far-infrared sauna. Far-infrared saunas directly warm the body, not the air around you. Consequently, your body is able to produce sweat at a much lower temperature than in a regular sauna and expel toxins through the exit organs, even the hair.

Two of the most important body regions for detoxification are the digestive system and the liver. There are two phases of detoxification for the liver. During Phase 1 the liver cells, assisted by an elaborate set of enzymes (P450 enzymes), convert fat-soluble (called lipophilic) toxins into water- soluble (hydrophilic). Why is this phase important? If these toxins remain in the system in a fat-soluble form without being neutralized, they can create problems in the body such as lethargy, headaches, mood issues, and digestive issues. The reason this occurs is because the toxins have a choice of being converted and cleared from the body (good!) or stored in fat cells (bad!). If you want to alleviate headaches, mood symptoms, and fatigue, the brain needs to be cleansed of any toxins that have accumulated there. Since 70% of the brain is comprised of fat, toxins love the brain because they have lots of areas to call home!

During Phase 1 of liver detoxification, this fat-soluble toxin is converted into an intermediate toxin through oxidation, reduction, and other enzymatic transformations. However, that isn't necessarily a safer form. Nutrients and various other substrates are needed for this to occur smoothly. If antioxidants such as Vitamin E are not present, these intermediate toxins can lead to free radical formation and increase toxicity to the body. During these times, this intermediate form can be more harmful than the fat-soluble form. The goal is to get this intermediate toxin through Phase 2 of liver detoxification. Before it goes through this phase, let's review what the body needs for this to happen.

Phase 1 Detoxification: Necessary Nutrients

- Vitamins B2 (Riboflavin), Vitamin B3, Vitamin B6, and Vitamin B12
- Folic Acid
- Glutathione
- Antioxidants (Vitamin C and Vitamin E)
- Magnesium
- Iron

From a dietary perspective, adding flax seeds and cruciferous vegetables such as broccoli and cauliflower are beneficial during Phase 1 of liver detoxification.

For those of you who take Fioricet or Fiorinal (brand names for the abortive medications containing Tylenol or aspirin/barbiturates and caffeine), I recommend exercising caution. These medications are notorious for inducing the Cytochrome P450 enzyme system. Why is that bad? If the Cytochrome P450 enzymes are induced without adequate antioxidant support, the body releases many toxic free radicals (with the conversion of fat-soluble toxins into intermediate compounds) into your system. Unless you are taking adequate nutrients or antioxidants, these medications can severely harm the body. In addition, medications such as Fioricet have three ingredients that have been reported to aggravate the liver: Tylenol, caffeine, and barbiturate all wrapped into one! I do not recommend taking these types of abortive medications unless there is no other abortive option. In the event that you are taking one of these medications, you must ensure that you are getting adequate nutrient, antioxidant, and liver detoxification support by using products that support these pathways (see Chapter 15 for more details).

Some foods may also trigger a toxic reaction. For example, if you drink large amounts of grapefruit juice while taking some of these medications, the body's enzyme system, which normally clears these meds out of the body, will be inhibited. The medication will remain in the body at higher levels, which can lead to increased side effects.

During my first year of practicing headache medicine, I recall being asked to create a chart of all medications and supplements that needed an optimally-functioning liver to be cleared or activated. I then created another chart that described how various medications and supplements can lead to an augmentation or inhibition of liver enzyme activity. It was quite a list — long enough to make your head spin!

Let me give you an example. In a situation where you are combining medications or over-the-counter pills, or if your liver is not able to clear toxins due to being overloaded, a 10 mg dosage of Prozac may feel as if you had taken a 20 mg dosage. This could lead to excess side effects such as nausea and fatigue.

After Phase 1 detoxification, the liver needs nutrients necessary for converting the fat-soluble toxins into water-soluble toxins, which will eventually be released through the kidneys, bile, and digestive tract. The kidneys filter wastes through the urine. If the liver does not have adequate stores of these nutrients, the body is unable to release the toxins during Phase 1. In addition, if there are too many toxins to clear, the liver may not be able to keep up with the process.

What happens during Phase 2 detoxification is quite fascinating. During this phase, your liver is busy taking fat-soluble toxins and converting them to water-soluble toxins so they can exit the body. If these water-soluble toxins cannot exit the body, they enter the lymphatic system and go back into circulation. This creates a greater risk to your tissues and cells. Other organs may attempt to jump in and help detoxify the system, such as the digestive organs and/or skin. But they can't do the amazing work of the liver; no organ can fill the shoes of the almighty liver!

During Phase 2, methylation and conjugation occur along with other enzymatic processes. The toxin is chemically modified so the body can release it.

Phase 2 Detoxification: Necessary Nutrients

- Methylated B vitamins

Milk thistle and methylated B vitamins, along with key nutrients such as magnesium, help augment this phase of liver detoxification. Calcium-D-Glucarate is also very beneficial in augmenting this phase of detoxification.

How Are These Toxins Removed from the Body?

Toxins accumulate in the fat and cell membranes (which are made up of fat) over a period of years, and removing these toxins is no easy task. It requires knowledge of your toxic load, utilization of appropriate nutrients and foods, and hydration to remove them from the body. Unfortunately, if this is not done appropriately, detoxification reactions such as migraines, nausea, constipation, and/or fatigue can easily occur.

Exercise and fasting are methods of detoxification used by many people. The use of nutrients, herbal supplements, and other Ayurvedic recommendations can also enhance the body's ability to detoxify and heal.

Curcumin, which is found in turmeric and gives it the beautiful yellow pigment, is used frequently to augment detoxification. This substance has the effect of removing carcinogenic substrates through Phase 2 of liver detoxification. It is a powerful spice and herbal supplement.

Because harmful substances generally exit the body through the colon, the digestive system plays an important role in the detoxification process. Toxins not cleared through the digestive system re-enter the circulatory system before being cleared through the liver. As you can see, the liver is quite busy filtering and clearing toxins from the environment, along with medications or over-the-counter products taken for pain. Consequently, the liver may become too overwhelmed to clear waste material from the colon. One cause of poor liver detoxification is chronic digestive issues.

The Ayurvedic Approach to Detoxification

In Ayurveda, one of the key principles to keeping the body in balance is to perform seasonal detoxifications. You have a unique doshic combination that can easily become imbalanced as the result of lifestyle and food choices, stress, and shifts in weather.

During the season change it's important to alter your routine, which is referred to in Ayurveda as *ritucharya* (seasonal routine). This is the time your body is preparing to correct imbalances through detoxification.

According to Ayurveda, each season has its own quality. During the summer months, when the sun is strong and the heat picks up, you feel more "heated." In Ayurveda, this is the Pitta time of the year. During this season, it's important to eat cooling foods such as watermelon and to drink beverages that are cooling by nature such as coconut water. In addition, it's essential to never skip lunch during the summer, which will aggravate Pitta fire.

During the transition from summer to fall, the body has to reset and readjust to the coming cooler weather. This is the time of the Vata dosha and feelings of restlessness, accompanied by gas and bloating. These are manifestations of the cold and dry wind state. This state can worsen with the winter months if the body is unable to adjust to the change of seasons. Performing an appropriate detoxification immediately prior to this time can help prevent or limit the manifestations of the symptoms.

During spring, the season of Kapha, the temperature increases and the air becomes moist, often with days of rain. Our dry, colder bodies now become warmer with more moisture. By specifically choosing foods that balance the dosha, the symptoms which often occur with season change can be reduced.

In addition, adding the herbal formula Triphala may prove to be quite useful (see Chapter 15 for details). This combination of three fruits (amalaki, haritaki, and bibhitaki) is one of the most powerful seasonal cleansers. It is particularly effective for cleansing the colon and it is very beneficial during any detoxification process. This formula is often taken daily, especially during the shift of seasons. In addition, adding digestive enzymes and spore probiotics can help the digestive system to fully clear out toxins during this time. Daily oil pulling, known Ayurvedically as *Gandusha*, is also a well-respected tool for detoxification. Our favorite is a combination of sesame oil, coconut oil, and turmeric, which is placed on the mouth and allowed to "bathe" the teeth and gums for 10-20 minutes as a daily morning routine. This simple technique has the effect of strengthening the gums and clearing bacteria from the mouth. I have been practicing this and find it allows me to feel more alert, along with helping my mouth feel clear and cleansed.

Now that we have discussed cleansing the mouth and colon, we can focus on choosing foods that support our dosha type and the specific time of the year. Generally, when it is cold outside, the Vata state tends to prefer warming foods. Choosing light, cooling, cleansing meals comprised of sprouted foods and salads can prove very beneficial to cooling the Pitta state during the summer.

During the change of season, it's important to not only change the types of foods consumed, but also alter the state of the food eaten in order to honor the change in your external environment. When foods aren't adjusted for the season, the dosha can easily become imbalanced. But when you take some time and truly listen to the request of your mind, you'll find that you crave foods that support balance.

Season	Elements	Ideal Food Choice
Summer	Fire and water Warm, humid	Sweet fruits, veggies Heavy foods (dairy) Cool foods and liquids Cooling spices: cilantro
Fall	Air and water Cool, wind	Heavy foods with spices Sweet fruits Root vegetables, soups Warming spices: cloves
Winter	Air and space Cold, dry	Heavier foods with spices Warming foods Soups, chili, well-oleated foods Warming spices: ginger
Spring	Earth and water Moist, warm	Light, cleansing, dry foods Salads, green drinks, berries Limit dairy Cleansing spices: cumin

Detox Your Mind *and* Body

As a neurologist with a background in psychiatry, I am always intrigued by the link between the brain and the mind. Whenever I see patients, I often ask when they last felt "optimal," or in perfect harmony. It is often distressing to hear my patients say that they have been experiencing the imbalance manifesting as migraines from a very young age. Patients also describe early symptoms of anxiety or social phobia during times of digestive distress. The question I always ask myself is, "Which came first — the imbalance of the mind or the imbalance of the body?" The beauty of Ayurveda, however, is that it really doesn't matter. The mind and body aren't treated separately; when it comes to healing one, the other is also being healed.

In terms of detoxification, the same rules apply. The thoughts that many of us experience can also create toxicity to the systems. Holding on to negative, angry thoughts or feeling emotionally blocked prevents the body from functioning optimally. During detoxification, it is also important to release and cleanse toxic thoughts from the mind. Many individuals use food to pacify stress and emotions, and this can increase toxins in the body. Utilizing various combinations of Ayurvedic herbals may help create a more balanced mind, which can help create emotional balance and harmony.

Now that you have learned about the importance of detoxification, take the following quiz to determine your own level of toxicity.

The Detox Quiz

1. **How many days per week do you exercise?**
   A. Daily
   B. 3-5 times per week
   C. 1-2 times per week
   D. Never
2. **How much alcohol do you drink per week?**
   A. Never
   B. 1-2 times per week
   C. 3-5 times per week
   D. Almost daily
3. **How many days per week do you eat out?**
   A. Never
   B. 1-2 times per week
   C. 3-5 times per week
   D. Almost daily
4. **How many bowel movements do you have per day?**
   A. Two or more bowel movements per day
   B. One bowel movement per day
   C. One bowel movement every 2-3 days
   D. One bowel movement every 1-2 weeks

5. How much water do you drink per day?

A. 8-10 glasses
B. 4-8 glasses
C. 2-3 glasses
D. 1 or less

6. Does your belly:

A. Lie flat with your pants
B. Rest a little over your pants
C. Hang over your pants

7. How many massages do you receive per year?

A. 6-12 per year
B. 3-6 per year
C. 1-3 per year
D. Never

8. Do you live in a community that is:

A. Rural
B. Suburban
C. Urban
D. Combination

9. What kind of cleaning products do you use?

A. Organic, Paraben-free always
B. Organic, Paraben-free most of the time
C. Organic, Paraben-free sometimes
D. Never organic or Paraben-free

10. When was your last detoxification?

A. In the last six months
B. About a year ago
C. 2-3 years ago
D. Never

Symptoms

11. Do you feel congested/heavy/blocked?

A. No
B. Mild, minor occasional neck or back stiffness
C. Moderate, often tight neck/back, congestion in throat
D. Severe, always tight neck/back, congestion in head/throat

12. Do you feel "awake" first thing in the morning?

A. Yes, clear immediately upon awakening
B. No, takes about 5-10 minutes to feel clear
C. No, takes about 15-30 minutes to feel clear
D. No, I really don't "wake up" for hours or maybe all day unless caffeinated!

13. Do you have a lack of motivation to get going?

A. Never
B. Yes, just recently and it only happens infrequently
C. Yes, for months and it happens a few days per week
D. Yes, for a long time and it is lasting for many hours per day

14. Do you feel fatigue/headaches and if so, when?

A. Never
B. Yes, only in the morning or afternoon and it's mild
C. Yes, for most of the day and it's moderate
D. Yes, for most of the day and it's moderate to severe

15. How would you describe your appetite?

A. I have a strong appetite and feel hungry at specific times: breakfast, lunch, and dinner.
B. I have a strong appetite and feel hungry only at 1-2 meal times per day — lunch and dinner, for example.
C. I have a moderate appetite and feel hungry only at one meal time per day.
D. I have a weak appetite and do not have hunger signals or a taste for foods.

Tally your answers. Calculate your totals by tallying up all of the responses to each letter, multiply by the digit listed below, and obtain your grand total:

A ________ x 1 = ____
B ________ x 2 = ____
C ________ x 3 = ____
D ________ x 4 = ____

Grand Total ________

15-20 points	Low toxin burden
21-30 points	Mild toxin burden
31-50 points	Moderate toxin burden
Greater than 50	High toxin burden

Based on the results, consider undergoing a one week to ten-day detoxification to jump-start the healing process and restore balance to your mind and body. In the next chapter, you'll learn about even more action steps you can take to improve your state of health and peace of mind.

CHAPTER 13

More Tools to Balance the Body and Mind

"Start where you are. Use what you have. Do what you can."
Arthur Ashe

In order to repair something — from a car to the state of your health — you need a toolbox. When I first started treating migraine patients in 2002, my toolbox contained only drugs and a few nutritional supplements I had learned about during my medical training or through personal inquiry. I had very little clinical experience utilizing diet, herbals, yoga, meditation, breath work, or other nutrients and herbals. I spent the first few years of my practice doing additional training in psychopharmacology (learning the mechanisms of how pharmaceutical drugs work in the body) and treating patients with a multitude of medications — from seizure medications to antidepressants — to quiet and calm the nervous system. While these medications did provide some relief, many patients felt unsatisfied and wanted more. Those patients whose symptoms responded to pharmaceuticals often returned with complaints of side effects. It was then that I decided to seek advanced training using complementary approaches.

I was pleasantly surprised to find that I could expand my toolbox to include more options for balancing the mind and body. As the number of available resources expanded, I suddenly realized that I needed a larger toolbox to contain all of the new tools available to help my patients heal. This entire book is my toolbox, and the following is a discussion of additional options that will help facilitate your ability to overcome migraines and other ailments.

Yoga

An Ayurvedic doctor once explained the relationship between yoga and Ayurveda by saying: "Ayurveda is the science and yoga is the practice of the science." They both encompass an understanding of how the body and mind work in concert, the impact that food has on the body, and the interconnection between the health of the body and the health of the mind. Yoga is used to create greater harmony in the body using a specific sequence of postures. Each sequence is based on the specific needs of the dosha. Yoga for the Vata dosha type focuses on settling the mind through relaxing postures. Yoga for the Pitta dosha type helps to cool off the body's excessive heat using calming and restorative postures. Yoga for the Kapha dosha type helps to create movement through invigorating yoga postures.

Meditation

The goal of meditation, which is a spiritual practice and not a religious practice, is to help you rediscover your body's own inner intelligence. Rather than attempting to force the mind to be quiet, the goal is to connect to the innate silence that already exists in order to create harmony and balance for your body and your mind. Meditation is also a potential resource for understanding your life's purpose, connecting with your intuition, and expressing yourself creatively.

I highly recommend that you establish a meditation practice based on your dosha, rather than attempting to adapt to a "one size fits all" practice. Vata dosha types will benefit from a meditation that aids in stillness. Pitta dosha types will benefit from a meditation practice that incorporates deep breathing. Kapha dosha types will benefit from guided visualization, contemplative questions, tai chi, or walking meditations.

Don't Be Afraid to Go There …

Now that you have taken time to learn about your dosha type and realize the effect an imbalanced dosha has on your whole system, take some time to delve into the mental aspects that may be holding you in an imbalanced state. Taking part in a mindfulness-based program such as yoga, meditation, or tai chi may help you fully understand where you are and where you need to be in terms of optimal mind health. Even herbals and nutrients may enhance your ability to delve further and deeper into your psyche. Do not be afraid; be open and accepting. Ask yourself the following questions, and do not rush to answer.

1) **Are you living the life you want? Do you have passion and purpose, or are you just doing what you have been told or are supposed to do? If your answer is "yes," was it your parental/family upbringing that led you to this life? If not, then how did this happen?**

2) **Are you always taking care of others, or do you make time for yourself? Do you have a hard time saying "no"? If your answer is "yes," why are you doing this and who are you trying to please?**

3) **Do you express your emotions well? Do you repress your emotions or become too emotional with various stressors? If your answer is "yes," in which dosha state do you find yourself imbalanced? Are you a perfectionist, worrier, or victim?**

4) **With whom do you surround yourself? Think of the five to ten people with whom you choose to spend the most time. Do they reflect you? Are they toxic (bringing you down with negativity) or are they supportive and uplifting?**

These are just a few of the questions that I think all of us should be asking ourselves. In this book we are unable to dedicate the time that is needed to truly delve into the complexities of the mind and how our parental upbringing, along with our nature, influences who we are and how we think. I highly recommend reading *When the Body Says No* by Gabor Mate, MD, for a further, deeper analysis of what happens when we do not speak our internal truth. Another excellent book to read is *You Can Heal Your Life* by Louise Hay, which delves into the mind behind the disease.

You've now gathered several important tools for restoring balance to your mind and body — an essential component in closing the case on your discomfort. But for some people, conventional medications are a necessary piece of the puzzle. Read on to learn about the most commonly-prescribed medications to treat migraine headaches and why I sometimes recommend their use.

CHAPTER 14

Common Medications Most Often Prescribed for Migraines

"Medicine is a science of uncertainty and an art of probability."
Sir William Osler

When I first began studying migraines, I was taught that migraines were a "neurovascular phenomena." According to what I learned, migraine evolution involved changes in the blood flow to the brain due to hypothalamic and brainstem shifts, leading to excitable neurons. If the pain continued, the nerves became inflamed and the blood vessels "leaked," thereby releasing more inflammatory proteins. I also was taught that there was often a "point of no return," or what was referred to in neurology lingo as "central sensitization." This occurred after headaches continued to the point that additional aspects of the nervous system were involved, making this attack very difficult to treat.

I spent an additional year after neurology training learning more about psychopharmacology (the study of the effects of drugs on mood, sensation, thinking, and behavior) so that I could fully understand how medications could be utilized for neurological conditions. I learned to prescribe medications for migraines that could stop the attacks (abortive medications) as well as medications that could prevent severe attacks (preventative medications). However, after working with patients over a period of three years, I was perplexed by the multiple headache types that could be experienced by an individual patient. On certain days, for example, the throbbing headache which included nausea seemed to be located on the right side of the head. At other times, the same person had a headache that was more aching in character and was located in the back of the head, in the neck region. The more I treated patients by strictly using pharmacology, the more uncertain and unsure I began to feel about the potential success of the treatment options I had at my disposal. The more I delved into integrative medicine, specifically Ayurveda, the more I understood the genesis of headache pain. I broadened my approach to incorporate both medications and supplements for various headache types.

Although my focus today is on helping patients make dietary and lifestyle changes that will improve their total well-being and alleviate symptoms, I recognize the importance of having the most effective tools of conventional medicine available when needed. This chapter provides an overview of the medications I most often prescribe, along with an explanation of how they work, demonstrating how I balance the best of the West with the best of the East in my treatment protocol.

Abortive Medications: Help Me When I Am in Pain!

Abortive medications are those used to "abort," or stop, attacks of pain. There are two types — specific and non-specific for migraines. Any medication that works on the serotonin nervous system is considered to be "specific." Serotonin is one of the most calming neurotransmitters of the brain. For some people, during a migraine the nerves become excitable. The brainstem along with the trigeminal nerve, which is responsible for sensation in the face and meninges (brain covering), can create the pain signals. Serotonin binds to certain receptors and quiets the signals. According to Dr. Michael Gershon, author of *The Second Brain,* "95 percent of the body's serotonin is found in the bowels."[57] Consequently, the body's storehouse of serotonin runs low and abortive medications are needed.

The main "specific" groups are known as the triptans. These include sumatriptan (Imitrex), frovatriptan (Frova), zolmitriptan (Zomig) and rizatriptan (Maxalt). Triptan medications have been the holy grail of migraine treatment, and most of them are effective and reliable. If triptans weren't available, I'm not quite sure how I would've been able to help my patients. Please try at least two or three different categories of triptans in different forms (e.g., nasel spray, patch, injectable) before determining the class is a "failure." It's when a triptan fails that I feel most perplexed about how to help manage acute pain.

Continued advances in the field of pharmacology have led to an increase in understanding which medications are most effective when migraines impact any of the seven serotonin subtypes 5-HT. I try to avoid prescribing narcotics and/or barbiturates due to the risk of dependency or addiction. In addition, research has found that these medications can potentially *increase* pain due to the impact they have on some of the body's serotonin receptors.[58]

Other medications that work on specific serotonin receptors (along with neurotransmitter receptors such as dopamine) are ergots, such as Migranal or DHE (dihydroergotamine). These have been available longer than the triptans. I prescribe Migranal to help break long cycles of migraines. It is beneficial because it doesn't lead to rebound.

There are also non-specific, abortive medications that don't seem to work directly on the "migraine center." These include muscle relaxants (Flexeril), anti-inflammatories (Aleve), narcotics (Vicodin), and steroids (Prednisone).

If the headache is milder, anti-inflammatories do seem to work well. One anti-inflammatory, diclofenac, is approved as an abortive for migraine. In more severe attacks, steroids or DHE seem to be very effective.

Preventative Medications: Help Me Prevent These Migraines from Happening Again!

There are three broad categories of preventative medications and many smaller categories.

Blood Vessel Regulators

The first options approved by the Federal Drug Administration (FDA) for migraine treatment were "blood vessel regulators." I use this name euphemistically so that patients don't think they have blood pressure issues. However, the truth is that these medications were first approved by the FDA to control high blood pressure (hypertension). Later, they were found to be helpful for other conditions. It is unfortunate that when it comes to new medication options, migraines are frequently on the back burner of research.

Beta-blockers are one of the categories of medications in this group approved for treatment of migraines. The FDA-approved choices are propranolol and timolol which, interestingly enough, seem to have an effect on serotonin activity.

Verapamil and Atacand are other medications also approved for hypertension but have generally been found to be helpful for certain headache conditions. Interestingly, Verapamil, which is a calcium channel blocker, seems to be most effective for patients who have a magnesium deficiency. When magnesium stores are replenished, Verapamil is usually no longer needed. I think that means that it may be beneficial for migraine patients to balance their magnesium levels first! For more information on this issue, read *The Magnesium Solutions for Migraine Headaches* by Jay Cohen, MD.

Neuromodulators

Neuromodulators was the second category approved by the FDA. These medications, which were approved to manage seizures, seem to have a quieting and calming effect on the nervous system. The most popular and FDA-approved medication in this category is topiramate (Topamax). This drug has gained popularity not only because of its effectiveness, but also because it helps with weight loss! It's one of the few preventatives that have this beneficial side effect.

Keep in mind that weight gain may be due to adrenal stress and/or toxin accumulation in fat cells, leading to metabolically-active fat cells. These active cells release inflammatory peptides that can be linked to the evolution of an intermittent migraine to a chronic, transformed migraine. According to a study about episodic migraine and obesity which included the influence of age, race, and sex, it was found that the odds of episodic migraine are increased in those with obesity, especially for people under the age of 50, white individuals, and women.[59]

It seems that topiramate works on multiple areas of the brain but is most effective in its role of blocking glutamate receptors, which quiet the brain. An interesting note: both magnesium and green tea also work to block glutamate.

Divalproex (Depakote) is also approved for migraine, but it comes with the potential side effects of weight gain, hair loss, and the elevation of liver enzymes. That's a high price to pay for improvement in migraines or moods. However, some patients have taken it because natural agents haven't been enough for their genetics or dosha type. It's important to always consider the risks and benefits of a medication versus a natural supplement.

Other neuromodulators are gabapentin (Neurontin), levetiracetam (Keppra), pregabalin (Lyrica), and oxcarbazepine (Trileptal). Although these drugs have not been well studied, they can be found to help alleviate pain in certain cases.

Other Medications

The third category of medications consists of FDA-approved drugs that impact but are not designated for the treatment of migraines.

Neurotransmitter Balancers

We have been trained to utilize the classification the FDA has given for these medications: antidepressants, antipsychotics, or anxiolytics. These labels often create a stigma for the patient since they are often not being prescribed for that purpose. In the event that I do prescribe one of these medications, it's due to low serotonin/norepinephrine levels (either genetics, fatigued adrenals, or poor production by the digestive system) or hormonal imbalance (caused by estrogen dominance).

While none of these medications have been designated by the FDA for treatment of migraines, they can be very effective in low doses when natural agents provide no relief. There are side effects: weight gain, loss of libido, and flattening of mood. I have even seen a depletion of nutrients, which also needs to be taken into account. For example, according to researchers, SSRIs (such as Prozac) can lead to low B vitamin levels.[60]

Botox Type A

You may be surprised to learn that despite my desire to make integrative medicine the foundation of my practice, there are many times when I have recommended Botox Type A for my patients. Why? Botox is an agent that I studied during my residency because I felt it offered a unique approach to treating patients suffering with pain.[61] Botulinum Toxin Type-A (onabotulinum toxin) has been approved by the FDA for use in treating chronic migraine since October 2010.

Botox Type A can lead to the reduction of migraines for three months after the injections are administered, due to its activity at the nerve ending.[62] It is believed to decrease the amount of CGRP (calcitonin gene-related peptide) released from the nerve ending. This peptide is considered a neuroinflammatory peptide responsible for inducing pain. With less neuro-inflammatory peptide release, the adrenals can reduce their release of cortisol and rest. I believe this is one of the best approaches available to not only arrest migraine pain but also provide a break for overstressed adrenals.

The Journal of the American Medical Association published a report regarding a study which found that patients with chronic migraines (15 or more/month) experienced some benefit from Botox injections.[63] Because Botox Type A is injected rather than ingested, there are limited effects on the digestive system, liver, and cognition.

I use Botox Type A to provide relief from chronic headaches. It serves as a bridge as patients begin utilizing integrative approaches such as supplements, nutrients, and changing their diets. This also limits the need for abortive medications. I think it's a win-win for many of my patients, especially now that most insurance coverage has expanded to cover its use for those with chronic migraines.

Ayurvedic Choices for Migraines

In Ayurveda, the Vata brain is the excitable brain with excess wind element. When treating patients according to the Ayurvedic headache model, I use calming medications such as valium, triptans, and/or muscle relaxants for a Vata-predominant headache. In terms of natural supplements, magnesium, GABA supplements, and/or 5HTP (the precursor of serotonin) may be wonderful options for this state.

The Pitta brain is the heated brain, which is prone to inflammation due to the augmented fire state. If the headache is occurring secondary to an excess of heat in Pitta, using anti-inflammatories and steroids may be the best option.

If headaches are due to excess Kapha, antihistamines and stimulant medications may be beneficial. Sometimes the brain is excitable, inflamed, and/or congested. In that case, multiple supplements and pharmaceutical agents from several categories may be the best way to alleviate the pain.

Additional Thoughts on Medications

Please keep in mind that medications should always be taken in small amounts and for short periods of time. Use caution when taking anti-inflammatory medications for headaches and pain over an extended period of time. Medications such as Advil, Excedrin migraine, Aleve, and steroids (Prednisone and Decadron) may lead to a decrease in healthy bacteria count in the intestinal tract and may lead to gastric erosions or ulcers. Use these medications cautiously or avoid them altogether.

Researchers have found a link between acid reflux and migraines.[64] Proton pump inhibitors, known as acid blockers, are often used when a patient is suffering with acid reflux. However, acid blockers can actually worsen the condition long term, even if there is short-term improvement in symptoms. The symptoms of reflux, which include burning and pain after meals, are often due to the incomplete digestion of foods and low stomach acid production. This condition, known as hypochlorhydria, is discussed in full in Dr. Alan Gaby's seminal work *Nutritional Medicine.* Low stomach acid production can be improved with supplementation of Betaine Hydrochloride (HCl) or a tablespoon of apple cider vinegar mixed in a quarter-cup of water during meals. Either of these helps to restore the proper acid levels in the stomach and maintain healthy GI function. They can reduce the sensation of reflux if hypochlorhydria is the cause.

According to Ayurveda, the symptom of reflux is the result of excess Pitta dosha type. Pitta often has been linked to migraines, too. Ultimately, the goal is to eat foods that balance this state and, when needed, take herbal and/or nutritional supplements that can heal the inflamed lining of the stomach.

In addition to conventional medications, I also recommend nutritional supplementation. Let's explore supplements in the next chapter, where you'll find details about numerous supplements and herbs that may be key to the mystery of restoring your health and well-being.

CHAPTER 15

Nutritional Supplements that Enhance the Quality of Your Health

"You must be the change you wish to see in the world."
Mahatma Gandhi

Functional medicine bridges the worlds of Western and Eastern medicine. Prescription medications are widely used because these are the tools that Western doctors were trained to employ. Medications and injectables do play an important role. However, the use of medication alone often doesn't allow the patient to determine the genesis of the symptoms or eradicate the root cause. For example, if digestion, weak adrenals, low hormones, or an imbalanced mind are the source of disease, conventional medicine will provide prescriptions for each imbalance. On the other hand, Eastern or alternative medicines such as Ayurveda seek to find the source of the imbalance first so that healing can begin and the symptoms can be eradicated. This approach takes more work, not only to understand but also to treat. However, in the long run, this approach will garner the greatest results. Using an integrative medicine approach allows the patient to benefit from a deep wellspring of knowledge and utilize the best strategies from both worlds.

Nutritional Supplements

Following is a list of recommended nutritional supplements and the benefits of taking them.

Probiotics

Many headache and chronic pain patients use steroids and non-steroidal anti-inflammatories for headache treatment. These medications have the potential to damage the balance of healthy bacteria in the intestinal tract, leading to digestive issues. This damage can create further nutritional deficiencies and cause headaches to worsen. Probiotics means "for life," and these microorganisms help maintain the immune system of the digestive tract and decrease the number of harmful bacteria and yeast. There are numerous medical, dietary, and lifestyle factors believed to disturb the bacterial balance in the colon, leading to an imbalance called dysbiosis. Factors include: antibiotic use; ingestion of environmental toxins; stress; eating meals inappropriate for your mind-body type; excess sugar and processed, low-fiber foods; and hormonal fluctuations.

When your intestinal tract is well-populated with healthy bacteria, the body is able to produce B vitamins (B1, B6, B9, Vitamin K); produce digestive enzymes; help absorb calcium, magnesium, and iron; and support the immune system. This is why probiotics and digestive enzymes are essential. The first step to strengthening the immune system, especially when food intolerances exist, is to begin taking probiotic supplements daily. The necessary dosage and number of strains of good bacteria is based on the needs of your digestive system.

Many doctors view probiotics as the first line of defense for immune system health. Remember, the lining of the colon is one of the main contacts your body has with the external environment. If you're exposed to toxins it's through your digestive tract, which has the unique role of regulating what is allowed into the body and what is excreted out of the body.

There are many types of probiotics on the market today, so choosing the right one can be confusing. Which "healthy bacteria" is the best? How many billions are enough? Are refrigerated probiotics better than non-refrigerated? Some probiotics are lower dosed, with fewer species. Are they as effective? The most important test you want your probiotic to pass is the ability to thrive in the digestive tract. Some doctors recommend a class of probiotics that form spores, which may be more stable in the digestive system. Research has found that probiotics containing bacillus spores survive the stomach acid intact. These spores then police the intestines, ridding it of unwanted bacteria, yeast, and fungi.

True probiotics are transient; I think of them as digestive housekeepers. They get into your bowel and competitively exclude pathogenic organisms, produce nutrients necessary for your body, and then move on to another host. While they are moving through the bowel they keep it healthy.

In Ayurveda, as in most other alternative therapies, we examine the health of the gut as an indicator for the health of the body. The key to vibrant health is a healthy digestive system.

Digestive Enzymes

I can still hear my mother's voice telling me, "Chew slowly, Trupti! Don't eat so fast or you will get a stomachache!" I never quite understood why I needed to slow down when I ate, or why she insisted that I chew my food 32 times before swallowing. Due to her insistence, at a very young age I envisioned a large, partially-chewed piece of broccoli getting stuck somewhere in my digestive system and causing pain. So, I did my best to listen and follow my mother's directions.

After finishing medical school, I began to contemplate those earlier conversations I had with my mother. I finally understood the scientific truth behind what I thought was simply my mother urging me to eat my food in a particular manner. Your body can only access the nutrients in the food if your digestive system is able to break it down and convert it into molecules that your cells, tissues, and organs can then use for metabolic functions and fuel. When you chew your food, breaking it into small pieces (and 32 chews is a good amount of time to break it down), your body releases enzymes to assist in the digestive process. It actually takes hours for your system to break down simple sugars, fatty acids, and amino acids so they are available for utilization by your body.

The three enzymes most essential to this process are amylase, protease, and lipase. Amylase is a digestive enzyme that targets the starches in food. Protease breaks down protein into its building blocks — amino acids. Lipase is the enzyme that breaks down dietary fats into smaller molecules, called fatty acids and glycerol.

There's an old adage that says, "Life is short. Eat dessert first." The truth is we do eat backwards. We *should* eat sweet foods first, followed by protein and fats, and then an astringent (like salad). The typical American diet, however, begins with salad and ends with dessert. This is actually contrary to the way the body naturally produces digestive enzymes.

The less processed the food, the more easily the body can extract it.

Consider making your diet at least 50-70% raw vegetables unless you have Vata symptoms, in which case raw may be hard to digest. Lightly sautéed may be the best option for you.

If laboratory tests show that your body is not producing enough enzymes, I recommend taking a digestive enzyme supplement to assist the body with this process.

Omega-3 Fatty Acids

Omega-3 fatty acids are essential fats your body needs for healthy nerve functioning, optimal brain function, heart health, and blood sugar stability. The body is unable to produce Omega-3 fatty acids, so they have to be consumed through food. There are two primary sources — oily fish is the source of EPA (eicosapentaenoic acid) and DHA (docosahexaenoic acid). Omega-3s are found in salmon, tuna, sardines, mackerel, and shellfish. Vegetarian sources of Omega-3 ALA (alpha-linolenic acid) come from such sources as walnuts; flaxseed; chia seeds; and extra virgin, cold-pressed organic olive oil. Omega-3 fatty acids help prevent systemic inflammation, which is the root cause of many chronic ailments and diseases, including headaches and cardiovascular disease.

What about Omega-6 fatty acids? Most of the Omega-6 oils in our diet come from prepared and processed foods and should be avoided, including canola, because this can lead to inflammation. However, it's important to add to your diet oils rich in natural Omega-6, including pumpkin seed, sunflower, evening primrose oil, borage oil, and hemp seed oil. These healthier forms of Omega-6 oils in moderation can help balance the brain and hormones.

Magnesium Glycinate and Citrate Chelate

Magnesium is one of the most beneficial and essential nutrients for the body's functional needs. It's a cofactor, involved in the activation of more than 300 enzymes in your body. Benefits of magnesium supplementation include improved sleep, decreased anxiety, relaxation of muscles, improved glucose uptake, improved bone health, and decrease of blood vessel constriction. Studies have documented the benefits of magnesium in migraine, especially menstrual cycle-related migraines.[65-68] The magnesium formula I recommend is combined with both citrate and glycinate. It is chelated, which makes it easier to digest, and is more tolerable, with very few side effects.

Vitamin D (cholecalciferol)

The fat-soluble Vitamin D3 is a hormone rather than a vitamin. Studies have documented low Vitamin D3 levels in migraine and links Vitamin D deficiency with headaches.[69-71]

Vitamin E (mixed tocopherols)

This vitamin is an antioxidant composed of eight fat-soluble compounds. It is linked to the prevention of Alzheimer's disease and can help boost your immune system along with improving the action of insulin, thus helping to regulate blood sugars. It's important to use the mixed tocopherols as found in nature. This form of Vitamin E has proven to be more beneficial and likely safer than the d-alpha or d-l alpha form found in most supplements.[72]

Vitamin B1 (thiamine)

Vitamin B1 helps the body adapt to stress and avoid adrenal burnout. It's necessary for energy production, carbohydrate breakdown, and thyroid hormone metabolism and is needed for proper nerve function. This vitamin can be depleted with the use of oral contraceptives.

Vitamin B2 or Riboflavin/Riboflavin 5 Phosphate

Vitamin B2, or riboflavin, is associated with most of the body's energy pathways. It's an essential vitamin for mitochondrial health, which is often found to be involved in migraine.[73] Vitamin B2 is needed to regenerate glutathione, the strongest antioxidant produced by the body. Vitamin B2 is also needed to convert other B vitamins into their active forms. Multiple studies have been conducted which demonstrate the benefit of Vitamin B2 in migraine patients.[74-78]

Vitamin B3 (niacin)

Vitamin B3, or niacin, is used in at least 40 chemical reactions in the body. This vitamin is well known for its potential cholesterol-lowering properties (it converts cholesterol to pregnenolone, a hormone that helps memory, amongst other things) and its role in mitochondrial energy production, which is often impaired in people with migraines. In addition, Vitamin B3 is necessary in the metabolism of tryptophan and serotonin and improves adrenal health. The study that showed its ability to decrease migraine is likely based on the above-mentioned properties.[79]

Vitamin B6 (pyridoxine)

Vitamin B6 is essential for detoxifying chemicals and is paired with more than 100 different enzymes. It's key to synthesizing several neurotransmitters, such as serotonin, which are linked to both insomnia and migraine.[80]

Vitamin B9 (folic acid)

Vitamin B9, or folic acid, is best known for its role in energy production. This vitamin detoxifies hormones such as estrogen, along with heavy metals, and is needed for the conversion of dopamine. Studies have shown folic acid to be helpful in the treatment of migraine, especially if associated with elevated homocysteine levels.[81]

Methylated Vitamin B12 (methylcobalamin)

This vitamin is synthesized by bacteria and may be found to be low in vegetarians, vegans, or people with digestive issues. Methylcobalamin is the active form of B12 and is useful in decreasing homocysteine levels, synthesizing SAM-e (which can be very helpful for mood disorders), and supporting adrenal health. This form of Vitamin B12 has also been linked to lowering glutamate levels, which have been linked to migraine, memory, and mood disorders.[82] Due to its ability to scavenge nitric oxide, Vitamin B12 has been found to be helpful in migraine in various studies.[83, 84]

CoQ10 (as ubiquinol)

This fat-soluble nutrient is responsible for producing energy for cells but must be used in the ubiquinol form. The ubiquinol form is the reduced, active, antioxidant form of CoQ10. Age makes it harder to convert CoQ10 to ubiquinol. This is one of the strongest antioxidants available, protecting cells from free radical damage. Remember that this nutrient can become depleted if one is taking a statin drug (cholesterol-lowering medication), certain blood pressure drugs, and antidepressant medications. This nutrient has been well studied for its benefits in reducing migraine headaches.[85-87]

Alpha-lipoic Acid

This nutrient is essential to good health. It reduces excess calcium and copper; recycles CoQ10, glutathione, Vitamin C, and Vitamin E; and helps insulin work more effectively. It also helps with cellular energy production and has been studied for its use in migraine.[88]

Petadolex (butterbur)

This plant has been used in Europe since 1972 for the prevention of migraine. It acts as an anti-inflammatory by inhibiting leukotrienes and histamine. It is also a muscle relaxant and pain reliever. In its natural state, however, butterbur also contains pyrrolizidine alkaloids (PAs), which are known to be liver toxins. However, the butterbur in the formula that I recommend has been proven to be free of PAs. Many studies have been published establishing the effectiveness of butterbur for treating migraines in adults and children.[89-91]

Green Tea Extract

Green tea, which comes from the Camellia sinensis plant, is one of the highest antioxidant teas known to humankind. The active component is EGCG, which has many health benefits. Many studies have been conducted showing its benefit in improving cholesterol, coronary artery disease and possibly obesity.[92, 93]

Milk Thistle

Silybum marianum is the active ingredient in the milk thistle plant. It has been used to treat both kidney and liver disease. This plant reduces blood sugar, increases production of glutathione, helps with gallbladder disease, reduces inflammation, and protects your liver from toxins.[94, 95]

5-HTP

5-HTP is an amino acid and the precursor to serotonin. This supplement is recommended to augment serotonin levels.[96] However, caution is recommended. This supplement should not be combined with triptans or serotonin reuptake inhibitors, which could increase the risk of serotonin syndrome. Serotonin syndrome symptoms, which can range from mild to severe, include shivering, diarrhea, muscle rigidity, fevers, and seizures.[97]

Ayurvedic Herbals to Balance Your Mind and Body

I am constantly amazed by the power of Ayurvedic herbals. Many of these herbs have been utilized for thousands of years to balance the body and the mind. Wonderful shifts in the system occur when these herbs are used in synergy and in optimal doses. Ayurvedic herbals provide a deeper level of treatment beyond replenishing nutrients and enzymes. They are often dosha-specific, so they address the root of the imbalance based on your individual and specific needs.

Turmeric (Curcuma longa)

Turmeric is yellow in color and is a strong anti-inflammatory, antioxidant, and natural antibiotic.[98-100] It improves intestinal flora and may have a positive effect on healing ulcers and reducing the symptoms of indigestion.[101-104] It supports the liver and may improve cholesterol profile.[105]

Brahmi (Centella asiatica)

This is the main herb used for brain health. Its name means "supreme knowledge." It can improve vitality, clarity, sense of calm, and focus. Brahmi clears toxins from the kidneys/blood; it can be a very calming, relaxing herb.[106, 107]

Shankhapushpi (Evolvulus alsinoides)

Shankhapushpi is used to promote healthy blood flow to the brain. It is known to calm the mind. Shankhapushpi is also known for correcting digestive issues.[108]

Jatamansi (Nardostachys jatamansi)

One of the best herbs for headaches, Jatamansi is often used to help memory, improve moods, eliminate insomnia, reduce abdominal pain, and decrease blood pressure. Jatamamsi also can have a calming effect and may improve liver function.[109]

Ashwagandha (Withania somnifera)

Ashwagandha is an adaptogenic, and it is considered to be the best rejuvenating and restorative herb. It helps to reduce the symptoms of overwork and promotes rest without drowsiness. It also clarifies and calms the mind and may balance hormones due to its adaptogenic effects on the adrenals, thus improving progesterone levels. It may also improve libido.[110, 111]

Amla (Emblica officinalis)

This fruit is very Pitta-pacifying and rejuvenating. Due to its high Vitamin C content, it's a powerhouse for strengthening the immune system. Amla appears to be especially effective for burning-type (inflammatory) pain. It also has been found to reduce the heat state found in migraine attacks.[112]

Tulsi (Ocimum sanctum)

Tulsi modulates the immune system and can help combat stress. It has anti-inflammatory and anti-carcinogenic properties.[113]

Guggul (Commiphora mukul)

Guggul cleanses toxins from the body, purifies the blood, rejuvenates tissues, and is a strong anti-inflammatory. It has the power to lower cholesterol and strengthen the thyroid.[114-116]

Gurmar (Gymnema sylvestre)

This is one of the most balancing herbs for blood sugar. Gurmar is very helpful for sugar cravings and weight management.[117, 118]

Triphala

Triphala is most effective for the digestive system. It is composed of three powerful herbs that have an important role in cleansing the blood and balancing the system. It is one of the most respected herbal combinations and has been used in India for more than 5,000 years.

Amalaki

Amalaki, which is very Pitta-pacifying, has very high Vitamin C content and can help the immune system. It works as a strong antioxidant and can improve digestion.[119]

Bibhitaki

Bibhitaki has a laxative effect, and it improves the digestive system. It also cleanses the respiratory tract. Bibhitaki has an antibacterial effect and can decrease congestion and cough. In addition, it has an adaptogenic effect which allows it to improve the immune system.[120]

Haritaki

Haritaki can improve nutrient absorption and digestion and help prevent gallstones. This herb helps to remove toxins and can help with weight loss. It pacifies all three doshas.[121, 122]

Choosing Supplements

Like conventional medications, the decision to use nutritional supplements and Ayurvedic herbs as part of your treatment is based on your specific needs and dosha type. When considering which supplements and herbs to include, it is important to evaluate factors such as biochemistry tests, lifestyle choices, dietary habits, and the frequency and intensity of migraines and other symptoms. Ultimately, the goal is to make sure that you're not only pain and symptom free, but on the road to correcting the biochemical and nutritional imbalances that further exacerbate the symptoms with which you struggle.

You've come a long way in understanding the mystery of your discomfort. You've collected clues, investigated options, and armed yourself with action steps. Now, you're ready to put the pieces of the puzzle together. Turn the page and prepare to close the case on pain and distress forever!

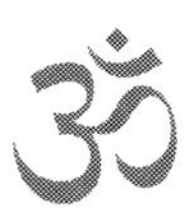

CHAPTER 16

Take the Next Step: The Plan

"A journey of a thousand miles must begin with a single step."
Lao Tzu

If you're like most people who will read this book, you picked it up because you were exasperated. You were in pain, your body felt older than your years, and you were frustrated that the concepts of balance and vitality seemed completely out of reach. You were looking for answers and you'd hoped that a physician who has treated and guided patients just like you might hold the clues to the mystery of your unhealthy body and mind.

Writing this book for you was an honor of great magnitude for me. I imagine you sitting on your couch or behind your desk, dog-earing pages and inserting Post-it notes (or inserting digital highlights if you are reading on Kindle). I hope you have found the insights to be inspiring. And I hope you know that taking the next step — translating these ideas into your own life — can be simple and profound.

While it was never my intent to solve the mystery of every mind — to profile every kind of patient who walks through the clinic doors seeking my help — it was my hope to share stories and information with you that might allow you to see your own health challenges through new eyes. Because, no matter how debilitating your pain or how unique your health situation, you are not alone.

After reading this book, you may feel a bit overwhelmed. You've learned a lot. Now, where to start? You'll overcome that sense of being overwhelmed by making a plan, and tackling it with confidence and vigor. Realize that this process is needed to heal your mind, thus improving your headaches or other symptoms you may be suffering with. This journey starts with understanding your physical body, then moving on to understanding your emotional body.

Are You Ready?

As you have learned by reading this book, your mind and body are connected. Where should you begin? Let's start with your comfort zone. Ask yourself if you are ready to address many systemic imbalances or just one. Do you want to continue to take medications and receive injections or use only natural supplements and yoga? Are you ready to make dietary modifications? Do you think you could handle seasonal detoxifications?

There are many avenues from which to choose. Do yourself a favor and choose one. You can start with something as simple as making lunch your biggest meal of the day or by adding a yoga class once a week. You can begin your day with a morning meditation. Just take one step toward taking charge of your health and well-being and — I promise you — you'll never look back.

A life free of symptoms is waiting for you. You deserve to feel optimal, be optimal and have a place in this world that allows you to give and receive as much happiness as possible.

Now it is up to you to take the next step. Remember that this first step may be one of many steps that lead you to your optimal state. The key is to take that step and start moving forward.

Consider sharing this book with your own medical team, like your primary care physician, as part of your plan. And remember that demystifying your health problems requires that you start listening — closely — to what your body is telling you. The human body is a magnificent system designed to alert you of danger by making you feel "ill at ease" so that you will sit up, take notice and change.

Please Keep in Touch!

I hope you will consider keeping in touch and sharing your health journey and successes with me and with the wider community. Here's how you can ensure that your learning continues and your health truly improves as a result of the investment of time you made in reading this book.

- Follow my monthly blog posts on *The Huffington Post.*
- Read my Zira Mind and Body blog, and subscribe to our newsletter at www.ZiraMindAndBody.com.

- Live in the Chicago area? Consider making an appointment or joining us for a wellness event, like a detox challenge or a healthy cooking class.
- Learn more about nutritional supplements at www.Shop.ZiraMindAndBody.com.
- Keep reading. Visit the Zira site and search for "Book List" to find out what health and wellness books I'm reading and recommending.
- Follow me on Facebook, LinkedIn and Twitter.
- Consider having me come speak to your corporation or other large audience. Learn more at www.DrGokaniSpeaks.com.

The optimal you awaits. And you deserve it.

Be well.

"If you can't fly then run, if you can't run then walk, if you can't walk then crawl, but whatever you do you have to keep moving forward."

Martin Luther King, Jr.

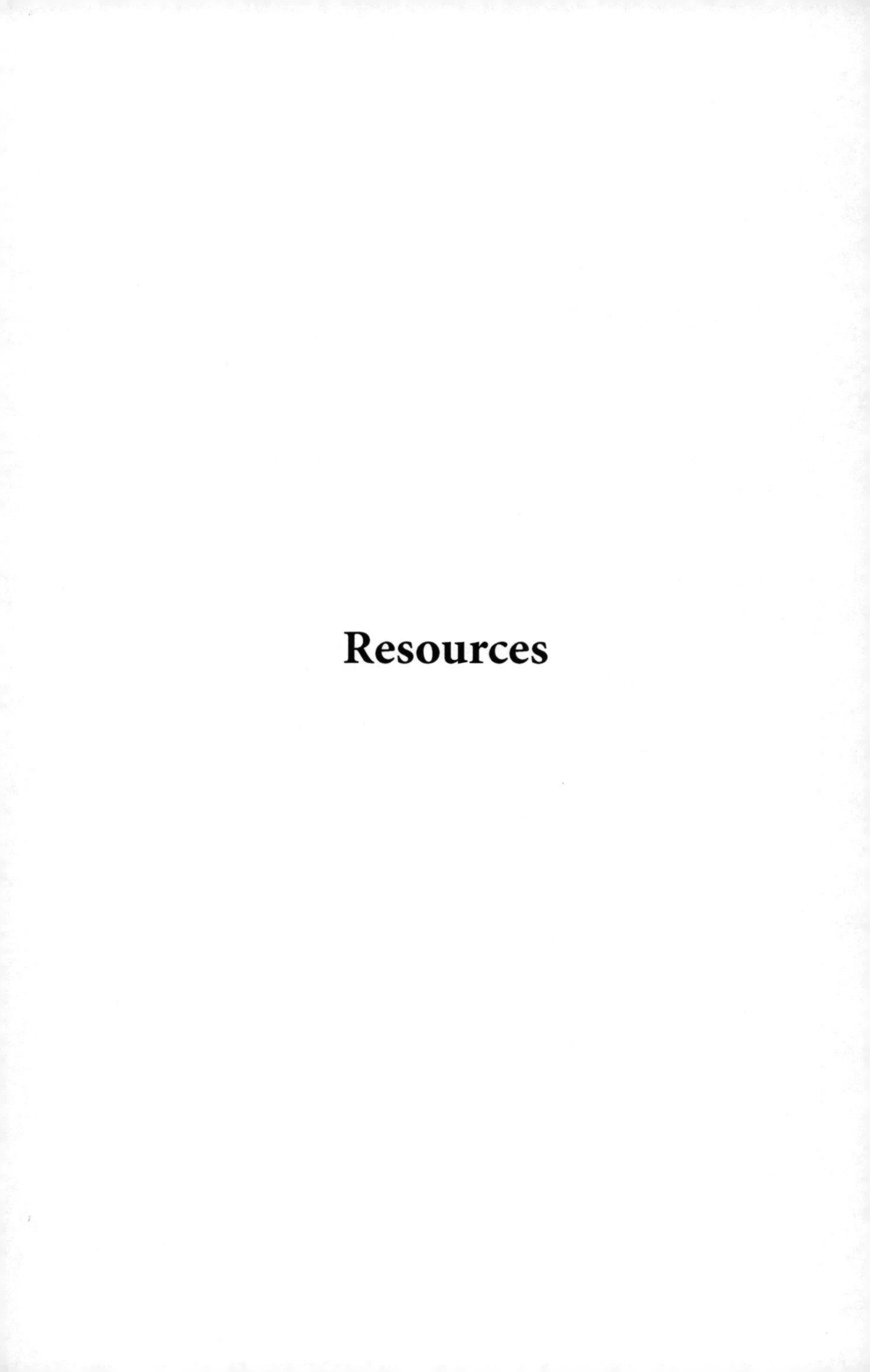

Resources

Appendix: Staging for Headache Sufferers

First Step: Determine Your Stage

Each stage involves lifestyle changes based on your dosha type and ability to make lifestyle modifications such as sleep, eating habits, etc.

Headache-specific Protocols

In Stage 1, many individuals are struggling with trying to manage their lives and function despite the severe pain. During this time, we often recommend traditional approaches to quiet the severity of pain, alongside approaches to balance the body. The program needs to be individualized for each patient.

Stage 1:

Severe attacks of pain, not responsive to abortive medications. These occur very frequently (more than 15 days per month)

- Consider Botox/preventative medications
- Address health issues of one system (digestion, adrenals, detox)
- Consider adding nutrients
- Consider seasonal detoxification
- Find better abortive options by combining medications, adding certain bio-identical hormones, adding injectables, and/or switching to patch forms of triptans (if not tried), etc.
- Incorporate an Ayurvedic, anti-inflammatory diet
- Add yoga and breathing exercises

In Stage 2, the frequency of the headache attacks is less, but each episode is moderate to severe in nature. During this stage, since the brain has the opportunity to rest between attacks, traditional approaches may not be needed and natural approaches likely have a higher chance of having their effects.

Stage 2:

Severe attacks of pain, abortives not helping, not very frequent

- Find better abortives to achieve pain freedom: 1st line, 2nd line, "rescue"
- Consider Sphenopalatine ganglion blocks, trigger point injections, steroids (limited doses)
- Work on two systems — digestion and adrenals/hormones/moods
- Add nutrients
- Incorporate an Ayurvedic, anti-inflammatory diet
- Add yoga and breathing exercises

In Stage 3, the frequency and severity of attacks are low. During this stage, one has the best chance of responding to dietary changes, lifestyle changes and natural approaches. Traditional medications may not be needed.

Stage 3:

- Infrequent attacks, responds well to abortives
- Add nutrients
- Consider nasya, turmeric/nutrients as abortives
- Work on two to three systems — digestion, hormones/adrenals, detoxification, moods
- Seasonal detox with fall/spring transition
- Yoga (1 hour/2 times per week), meditation (15 minutes daily), and cardio (30 minutes/one time per week)

References

[1] Cau, C., "The Alice in Wonderland Syndrome," National Center of Biotechnology Information, http://www.ncbi.nlm.nih.gov/pubmed/10767914.

[2] Krishan, Sonica, *Healing Through Ayurveda* (New Delhi, India: Rupa Publications, 2011).

[3] *Ibid.*

[4] Katic, B.J., Golden, W., Cady, R.K., Hu, X.H., "GERD Prevalence in Migraine Patients and the Implication for Acute Migraine Treatment," *Journal of Headache Pain*, 2009 Feb;10(1):35-43. doi: 10.1007/s10194-008-0083-1. Epub 2008 Nov 14. Center for PharmaceuticalHealth Services Research, Temple University School of Pharmacy.

[5] Rothenberg, Stuart, "Understanding the Six Stages of Disease," http://www.mapi.com/ayurvedic-knowledge/immunity/ayurvedic-understanding-of-disease.html.

[6] Dzugan, Sergey, MD, PhD, *The Migraine Cure*, pp. 33-34.

[7] Hyman, Mark, MD, *The Blood Sugar Solution*, pp. 4, 196-200.

[8] Wald, Michael B., MD, DC, *Encyclopedia of Nutritional Interpretation of Blood Tests*, p. 152.

[9] Smith, Pamela Wartian, MD, MPH, *HRT: The Answers. A Concise Guide to Solving the Hormone Replacement Therapy Puzzle*, p. 32.

[10] Holick, Michael F., PhD, MD, *The Vitamin D Solution: A 3 Step Strategy to Cure Our Most Common Health Problems*, pp. 3-22, 40.

[11] *Ibid.*, pp. 21-22, 64-68, 133.

[12] *Ibid.*, p. 40.

[13] Arem, Ridha, MD, *The Thyroid Solution*, pp. 239, 259.

[14] *Ibid.*, pp. 54-55.

[15] Rothenberg, Ron, MD, "Bio-identical Training Seminar," A4M.

[16] *Ibid.*

[17] Arem, Ridha, MD, *The Thyroid Solution*, pp. 237-238.

[18] Dzugan, Sergey, MD, PhD, *The Migraine Cure*, pp. 60-61.

[19] Smith, Pamela Wartian, MD, MPH, *HRT: The Answers. A Concise Guide to Solving the Hormone Replacement Therapy Puzzle*, pp. 46-51.

[20] Rothenberg, Ron, MD, "Bio-identical Training Seminar," A4M.

[21] *Ibid.*

[22] Arem, Ridha, MD, *The Thyroid Solution*, pp. 242-250.

[23] Dzugan, Sergey, MD, PhD, The Migraine Cure, pp. 60-61.

[24] Lang, Janet, DC, "Balance Female Hormones Naturally: The Essential Physiology & Principles," Seminar, January 2008.

[25] Speroff, Leon, and Fritz, Mark, Clinical Gynecologic Endocrinology and Infertility, 7th Ed. Lippincott Williams & Wilkins, 2005 p. 39

[26] Dzugan, Sergey, MD, PhD, *The Migraine Cure*, pp. 65-68.

[27] Smith, Pamela Wartian, MD, MPH, *HRT: The Answers. A Concise Guide to Solving the Hormone Replacement Therapy Puzzle*, pp. 29-34.

[28] *Ibid.*, pp. 17-20.

[29] Dzugan, Sergey, MD, PhD, *The Migraine Cure*, pp. 72-73.

[30] Institute of Functional Medicine, Training Course, 2012.

[31] Wright, Jonathan V., MD, and John Morgenthaler, *Natural Hormone Replacement for Women Over 45*, pp. 25, 71-72.

[32] Smith, Pamela Wartian, MD, MPH, *HRT: The Answers. A Concise Guide to Solving the Hormone Replacement Therapy Puzzle*, pp. 83-84.

[33] Institute of Functional Medicine, Training Course, 2012.

[34] Pacholok, RN, BSN, and Jeffrey J. Stuart, DO, *Could it Be B12*?, pp. 12, 18-21, 195-198.

[35] Hyman, Mark, MD, *The Blood Sugar Solution*, pp. 106-109.

[36] Keller, Daniel M., "Migraine Attacks Shortened by Diamine Oxidase Supplements," http://www.medscape.com/viewarticle/811920, Oct. 1, 2013.

[37] *Ibid.*

[38] Weil, Andrew, MD, "What is Leaky Gut?" (first published online), http://www.drweil.com/drw/u/QAA361058/what-is-leaky-gut.html.

[39] McEwen, Bruce S., "Protection and Damage from Acute and Chronic Stress: Allostasis and Allostatic Overload and Relevance to the Pathophysiology of Psychiatric Disorders," *Annals of the New York Academy of Sciences*, 1032: 1–7. doi: 10.1196/annals.1314.0012.

[40] *Ibid.*

[41] Wilson, James L., *Adrenal Fatigue: The 21st Century Stress Syndrome* (Petaluma, CA: Smart Publications, 2001), pp. 52-53.

[42] Cass, Hyla, MD, *Supplement Your Prescription: What Your Doctor Doesn't Know About Nutrition.*

[43] Lad, Vasant, *Ayurveda: The Science of Self-healing* (Wilmot, Wisconsin: Lotus Press, 1984), p. 19.

[44] *Ibid., p. 31.*

[45] Lad, Vasant, *Ayurvedic Perspectives on Selected Pathologies*, 2nd Edition (Albuquerque, NM: Ayurvedic Press, 2012), pp. 171-172.

[46] Lad, Vasant, *Ayurveda: The Science of Self-healing* (Wilmot, Wisconsin: Lotus Press, 1984), p. 32.

[47] Bellini, Bendetta, Arruda, Marco, Cescut, Alessandra, Saulle, Cosetta, Persico, Antonello, Carotenuto, Marco, Gatta, Michela, Nacinovich, Renata, Piazza, Fausta Paola, Termine, Cristiano, Tozzi, Elisabetta, Lucchese, Franco and Guidetti, Vincenco, *The Journal of Headache and Pain* 2013, 14:79, doi:10.1186/1129-2377-14-79.

[48] Krishan, Sonica, *Healing Through Ayurveda*, pp. 34-36.

[49] Bigal, M.E., Kurth, T., Santanello, N., Buse, D., Golden, W., Robbins, M., and Lipton, R.B., "Migraine and Cardiovascular Disease, A Population Study," *Neurology* (first published online), http://www.neurology.org/content/74/8/628.short.

[50] "What is Childhood Obesity?," American Heart Association, (first published online), http://www.heart.org/HEARTORG/GettingHealthy/HealthierKids/ChildhoodObesity/Whatis-childhood-obesity_UCM_304347_Article.jsp.

[51] Moss, Michael, "The Extraordinary Science of Addictive Junk Food," *The New York Times Magazine,* February 20, 2013. Accessed online: http://www.nytimes.com/2013/02/24/magazine/the-extraordinary-science-of-junk-food.html.

[52] Yarema, Thomas , Rhoda, Daniel, and Brannigan, Johnny, *Eat-Taste-Heal: An Ayurvedic Cookbook for Modern Living* (Whitefish, MT: Five Elements Press, 2006), pp. 41-42.

[53] Darbre, Philippa D., Harvey, Philip W., "Paraben esters: Review of recent studies of endocrine toxicity, absorption, esterace and human exposure, and discussion of potential human health risks," *Journal of Applied Toxicology* 2008, 28: 561-578.

[54] *Ibid.*

[55] Blumberg, Bruce, "What Do We Know About Obesogens?," htp://ehp.niehs.nih.gov/julypodcast/.

[56] Holtcamp, Wendee, "Obesogens: An Environmental Link to Obesity," *Environmental Health Perspectives*, http://www.ncbi.nlm.nih.gov/pmc/articles/PMC3279464/.

[57] Gershon, Michael, as quoted by writer Adam Hadhazy, "Think Twice: How the Gut's 'Second Brain' Influences Mood and Well-Being," *Scientific American*, February 12, 2010, http://www.scientificamerican.com/article/gut-second-brain/.

[58] Lee, Marian, Silverman, Sanford, Hansen, Hans, Patel, Vikram and Manchikami, Laxmaiah, "A Comprehensive Review of Opiod-Induced Hyperalgesia," Pain Physician 2011: 14:145-161, ISSN 1533-3159, accessed online, http://www.integration.samhsa.gov/pbhci-learning-community/opioid-induced_hyperalgesia_article.pdf.

[59] Peterlin, B. Lee, et al, "Episodic migraine and obesity and the influence of age, race, and sex," *Neurology* (first published online), http://www.neurology.org/content/early/2013/09/11/WNL.0b013e3182a824f7.short.

[60] Cass, Hyla, MD, *Supplement Your Prescription: What Your Doctor Doesn't Know About Nutrition*, p. 117.

[61] *American Journal of Pain Management*, July 2002, Vol. 12, pp. 79-85.

[62] *Ibid.*

[63] Jackson, Jeffrey L., et al., "Botulinum Toxin A for Prophylactic Treatment of Migraine and Tension Headaches in Adults," *Journal of the American Medical Association*, http://jama.jamanetwork.com/article.aspx?articleid=1148201.

[64] Katic, B.J., Golden, W., Cady, R.K., Hu, X.H., "GERD prevalence in migraine patients and the implication for acute migraine treatment," *Journal of Headache Pain,* 2009 Feb;10(1):35-43. doi: 10.1007/s10194-008-0083-1. Epub 2008 Nov 14. Center for Pharmaceutical Health Services Research, Temple University School of Pharmacy.

[65] Weaver, K., "Magnesium and migraine," *Headache*, 1990;30:168.

[66] Peikert A, Wilimzig C, Kohne-Volland R. Prophylaxis of migraine with oral magnesium: results from a prospective, multi-center, placebo-controlled and double-blind randomized study. *Cephalalgia*, 1996;16:257–263.

[67] Facchinetti, F., Sances, G., Borella, P., et al, "Magnesium prophylaxis of menstrual migraine: effects on intracellular magnesium," *Headache*, 1991;31: 298–304.

[68] Wang, F., Van Den Eeden, S.K., Ackerson, L.M., et al., "Oral magnesium oxide prophylaxis of frequent migrainous headache in children: a randomized, doubleblind, placebo-controlled trial," *Headache*, 2003;43:601-610.

[69] Prkash, S., Mehta, N.C., Dabhi, A.S., Lakhani, O., Khilari, M.J., *Headache Pain*. 2010 Aug; 11(4): 301-7. Epub 2010 May 13. "The prevalence of headache may be related with the latitude: a possible role of Vitamin D insufficiency?"

[70] Thys-Jacobs, S., "Alleviation of migraines with therapeutic vitamin D and calcium," *Headache*, 1994; 34: 590-592.

[71] Thys-Jacobs, S, "Vitamin D and calcium in menstrual migraine," *Headache*, 1994; 34: 544-546.

[72] Smith, Pamela Wartian, MD, MPH, *What You Must Know about Vitamins, Minerals, Herbs & More: Choosing the Nutrients That are Right for You*, pp. 24-27.

[73] *Ibid.*, pp. 33-34.

[74] Smith, C.B., "The role of riboflavin in migraine," *Canadian Medical Association*, J1946; 54: 589-591.

[75] Gordon, L., "Riboflavin in migraine," *British Medical Journal*, 1956; 2: 550-551.

[76] Schoenen, J., Lenaerts, M., Bastings, E., "High-dose riboflavin as a prophylactic treatment of migraine: results of an open pilot study. *Cephalalgia* 1994; 14: 328-329.

[77] Schoenen, J., Jacquy, J., Lenaerts, M., "Effectiveness of high-dose riboflavin in migraine prophylaxis: A randomized controlled trial," *Neurology*, 1998; 50: 466-470.

[78] Boehnke, C., Reuter, U., Flach, U., et al., "High-dose riboflavin treatment is efficacious in migraine prophylaxis: an open study in a tertiary care centre," *European Journal of Neurology*, 2004; 11: 475-477.

[79] Hall, J.A., "Enhancing niacin's effect for migraine," *Cortlandt Forum*, 1991: July 1: 46.

[80] Smith, Pamela Wartian, MD, MPH, *What You Must Know about Vitamins, Minerals, Herbs& More: Choosing the Nutrients That are Right for You*, pp. 39-41.

[81] Di Rosa, G., Attina, S., Spano, M., et al., "Efficacy of folic acid in children with migraine, hyperhomocysteinemia and MTHFR polymorphisms," *Headache*, 2007; 47: 1342-1344.

[82] Lea, R., Colson, N., Quinlan, S., et al., "The effects of vitamin supplementation and MTHFR ~C677T genotype on homocysteine-lowering and migraine disability," *Pharmacogenet Genomics*, 2009; 19: 422-428.

[83] Akaike, A., Tamura, Y., Sato, Y., Yokota, T., "Protective effects of a vitamin B12 analog, methylcobalamin, against glutamate cytotoxicity in cultured cortical neurons," *European Journal of Pharmacology*, 1993 Sep 7; 241(1): 1-6.

[84] Van der Kuy, PHM, Merkus, FWHM, Lohman, JJHM, et al., "Hydroxocobalamin, a nitric oxide scavenger, in the prophylaxis of migraine: an open, pilot study," *Cephalalgia*, 2002; 22: 513-519.

[85] Hershey, AD, Powers, SW, Vockell, ALB, et al., "Coenzyme Q10 deficiency and response to supplementation in pediatric and adolescent migraine," *Headache*, 2007; 47: 73-80.

[86] Rozen, TD, Oshinsky, ML, Gebeline, CA, et al., "Open label trial of coenzyme Q10 as a migraine preventive," *Cephalalgia*, 2002; 22: 137-141.

[87] Sandor, PS, Di Clemente, L, Coppola, G, et al., "Efficacy of coenzyme Q10 in migraine," *Neurology*, 2005, Feb 22; 64(4): 713-5.

[88] Magis, D, Ambrosini, A, Sandor, P, et al., "A randomized double-blind placebo controlled trial of thioctic acid in migraine prophylaxis," *Headache*, 2007; 47: 52-57.

[89] "Effectiveness of Petasites hybridus preparations in the prophylaxis of migraine: a systematic review," *Phytomedicine*, 2006.

[90] Anon, International team of researchers find herbal extract to be effective in preventing migraine (press release). Bronx, NY: Albert Einstein College of Medicine. Dec. 28, 2004.

[91] Lipton RB, Gobel H, Einhaupl KM, Wilks K, and Mauskop A. Petasites hybridus root (butterbur) is an effective preventive treatment for migraine. *Neurology*, Dec. 28, 2004; 63: 2240-2244

[92] "Green Tea," Medline Plus, http://www.nlm.nih.gov/medlineplus/druginfo/natural/960.html.

[93] *The One Earth Herbal Sourcebook. Everything You Need to Know About Chinese, Western, and Ayurvedic Herbal Treatments,* Alan Keith Tillotson, PhD, A.H.G, D.Ay, pp. 213-214.

[94] *Ibid.*, pp. 165-167.

[95] Smith, Pamela Wartian, MD, MPH, *What You Must Know About Vitamins, Minerals, Herbs & More: Choosing the Nutrients That are Right for You*, p. 176.

[96] *Ibid.*, pp. 128-129.

[97] Gaby, Alan, MD, "Serotonin syndrome symptoms, which range from mild to severe, include shivering, diarrhea, muscle rigidity, fevers and seizures," *A-Z Guide to Drug-Herb-Vitamin Interactions*, p. 237.

[98] Arora R.B, Kapoor, V., Basu, N., Jain, A.P., "Anti-inflammatory studies on Curcuma longa (turmeric)," *Indian Journal of Medical Research,* 1971; 59: 1289-95.

[99] Garodia, P., Ichikawa, H., Malani, N., Sethi, G., Aggarwal, B.B., "From ancient medicine to modern medicine: Ayurvedic concepts of health and their role in inflammation and cancer," *J Soc Integr Oncol,* 2007; 5: 25-37.

[100] Selvam, R., Subramanian, L., Gayathri, R., Angayarkanni, N., "The anti-oxidant activity of turmeric (Curcuma longa), *Journal of Ethnophramacology,* 1995; 47: 59-67.

[101] Gilani, A.H., Shah, A.J., Ghayur, M.N., Majeed, K., Pharmacological basis for the use of turmeric in gastrointestinal and respiratory disorders.

[102] Kositchaiwat, C., Kositchaiwat, S., Havanondha, J., "Curcuma longa Linn. in the Treatment of Gastric Ulcer Comparison to Liquid Antacid: A Controlled Clinical Trial.," *Journal of the Medical Association of Thailand,* 1993; 76: 601-5.

[103] Mahady, G.B., Pendland, S.L., Yun, G., Lu, Z.Z., Turmeric (Curcuma longa) and curcumin inhibit the growth of Helicobacter pylori, a group 1 carcinogen.

[104] Prucksunand, C., Indrasukhsri, B,, Leethochawalit, M., Hungspreugs, K., "Phase II clinical trial on effect of the long turmeric (Curcuma longa Linn.) on healing of peptic ulcer," *Southeast Asian J Trop Med Public Health*, 2001; 32: 208-15.

[105] Tillotson, Alan Keith, PhD, *The One Earth Herbal Sourcebook: Everything You Need to Know About Chinese, Western, and Ayurvedic Herbal Treatments*, pp. 220-221.

[106] Gohil, Kashmira J., Patel, Jagruti A., and Gajjar, Anuradha K., "Pharmacological Review on *Centella asiatica:* A Potential Herbal Cure-all," *Indian J Pharm Sci,* 2010 Sep-Oct; 72(5): 546-556.

[107] "Centella Asiatica," Earth Medicine Institute, http://earthmedicineinstitute.com/more/library/medicinal-plants/centella-asiatica/.

[108] Lad, Vasant, *Ayurvedic Herbology Student Handbook*, pp. 82-83.

[109] *Ibid.*, pp. 64-65.

[110] Tillotson, Alan Keith, PhD, *The One Earth Herbal Sourcebook: Everything You Need to Know About Chinese, Western, and Ayurvedic Herbal Treatments,* pp. 100-102.

[111] Lad, Vasant, *Ayurvedic Herbology Student Handbook*, pp. 32-33.

[112] Tillotson, Alan Keith, PhD, *The One Earth Herbal Sourcebook: Everything You Need to Know About Chinese, Western, and Ayurvedic Herbal Treatments*, pp. 97-98.

[113] *Ibid.*, pp. 218-220.

[114] Frawley, David, and Lad, Vasant, *The Yoga of Herbs: An Ayurvedic Guide to Herbal Medicine*, pp. 172-174.

[115] Tillotson, Alan Keith, PhD, *The One Earth Herbal Sourcebook: Everything You Need to Know About Chinese, Western, and Ayurvedic Herbal Treatments*, pp. 146-148.

[116] Smith, Pamela Wartian, MD, MPH, *What You Must Know About Vitamins, Minerals, Herbs & More: Choosing the Nutrients That are Right for You*, p. 183.

[117] Tillotson, Alan Keith, PhD, *The One Earth Herbal Sourcebook: Everything You Need to Know About Chinese, Western, and Ayurvedic Herbal Treatments*, pp. 149-150.

[118] Smith, Pamela Wartian, MD, MPH, *What You Must Know About Vitamins, Minerals, Herbs & More: Choosing the Nutrients That are Right for You*, pp. 183-184.

[119] Tillotson, Alan Keith, PhD, *The One Earth Herbal Sourcebook: Everything You Need to Know About Chinese, Western, and Ayurvedic Herbal Treatments.*

[120] Lad, Vasant, *Ayurvedic Herbology Student Handbook*, pp. 40-41.

[121] Frawley, David, and Lad, Vasant, *The Yoga of Herbs: An Ayurvedic Guide to Herbal Medicine*, pp. 174-175.

[122] Tillotson, Alan Keith, PhD, *The One Earth Herbal Sourcebook: Everything You Need to Know About Chinese, Western, and Ayurvedic Herbal Treatments*, pp. 150-152.

Index

Acknowledgements

I would like to thank the following people whose love and support made it possible for this book to exist: my husband Binal and my wonderful children, Ariya and Arman, who have taught me to be present, laugh, and stay in the moment and who also patiently endured years of my focusing on my passion, often with the sacrifice of family time; my parents and my in-laws who have helped raise my children and provide many lovely meals to nourish my family; my siblings, Dipti and Reena, and sister-in-law Shruti who have all supported me through this mission of evolving and learning and never questioned my decisions; my dear friends who allowed me to share the stress of balancing work, life, and motherhood and comforted me with kind words; my wonderful book editors Jeri Love, Nicole Yugovich, and Michelle Frieler, who gave my words more meaning, passion, and my authentic voice; my talented marketing, editing, and illustrations team at Silver Tree Communications, Kate Colbert, Lynn Granstrom, and Amy Bilello, who diligently put great effort into helping me create a book that matched my vision and worked tirelessly to get this mission accomplished; my team and partners at the office: Jackie, who has stood by and supported me; Tom and Ingrid, who are the perfect combination of fabulous energy, and inspire me to do something bigger and better with my work; and Ann, Whitney, Meg, Clare, and the rest of the team, for your hard work, awesome suggestions, and positive teamwork; and our lovely dog, Blue, who always greets me with love and joy. Last, but not least, I would like to thank my inner divine energy, and the energy of above, in alignment with my intuition, which has guided me to make the right choices, though many were not easy, and to create a life of meaning and purpose.

About the Author

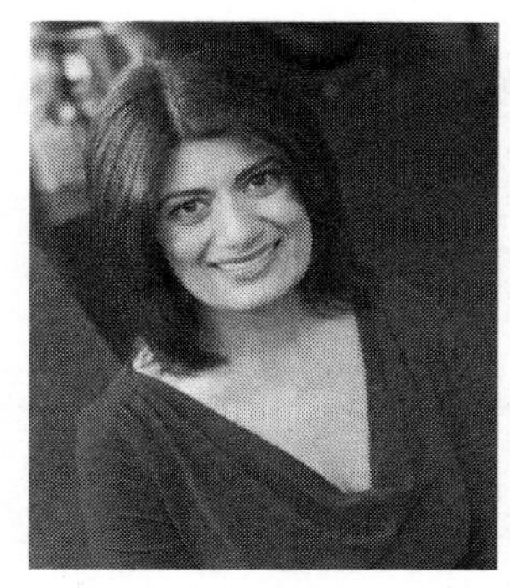

Trupti Gokani, MD, is an award-winning, board-certified neurologist best known for her innovative and integrative approach to treating headache pain. Her unique melding of modern medicine and ancient wisdom has enabled her to establish a thriving private practice along Chicago's North Shore. When not in the clinic, Dr. Gokani dedicates her time and significant insights to helping the wider community understand how to feel optimal, through a deeper appreciation of the mind-body connection.

Dr. Gokani is a sought-after trainer and speaker, having lectured extensively in the field of neurology and psychiatry, specifically regarding headaches, mood disorders, insomnia, adrenal fatigue, hormonal issues and adult attention deficit disorder (ADD). She has spoken at the American Headache Society, the Midwest Pain Society, the American Academy of Neurology, and the American Psychiatric Society. Her work — on topics ranging from Botox efficacy and safety, to the prevalence of bipolar disorder in cluster headache patients — has been published in such esteemed journals as the *American Journal of Pain Management.* She has also published articles pertaining to food allergies and headaches, along with the Ayurvedic approach to migraine, in the well-regarded *Journal of Headache.*

Dr. Gokani is a Magna Cum Laude (Biology/Economics) graduate from the University of Illinois at Urbana-Champaign, received her Doctor of Medicine (MD) degree from the University of Illinois at Chicago, and completed her training in Neurology at the University of Illinois at Chicago (where she was Chief Resident during her final year).

Dr. Gokani has been featured on The Dr. Oz Show, is a blogger for *The Huffington Post,* and is part of a forthcoming documentary on Ayurveda. She lives in Glenview, IL, with her supportive husband, two lovely children, and beautiful dog Blue. This is her first book.

Enjoy a Special Gift from Dr. Gokani

Please enjoy a complimentary copy of *Lose Weight and Feel Great: The Ayurvedic Way* – a healthful guide that was compiled to give readers of *The Mysterious Mind* an understanding of how the Ayurvedic diet compares to other types of diets. This book will delve into the Ayurvedic diet and compare it to other common diets. You will then have access to some of Dr. Gokani's special healing recipes, with tips on each ingredient, to help you begin the journey of balancing your mind and body with food and spices.

Download your copy today at www.ZiraMindAndBody.com/delicious.

42577114R00101

Made in the USA
San Bernardino, CA
06 December 2016